MW01127313

Triple-Negative Breast Cancer

Antoinette R. Tan
Editor

Triple-Negative Breast Cancer

A Clinician's Guide

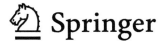 Springer

Editor
Antoinette R. Tan, MD, MHSc, FACP
Department of Solid Tumor Oncology and Investigational Therapeutics
Levine Cancer Institute
Carolinas HealthCare System
Charlotte, NC
USA

ISBN 978-3-319-69979-0   ISBN 978-3-319-69980-6   (eBook)
https://doi.org/10.1007/978-3-319-69980-6

Library of Congress Control Number: 2017963257

© Springer International Publishing AG 2018
This work is subject to copyright. All rights are reserved by the Publisher, whether the whole or part of the material is concerned, specifically the rights of translation, reprinting, reuse of illustrations, recitation, broadcasting, reproduction on microfilms or in any other physical way, and transmission or information storage and retrieval, electronic adaptation, computer software, or by similar or dissimilar methodology now known or hereafter developed.
The use of general descriptive names, registered names, trademarks, service marks, etc. in this publication does not imply, even in the absence of a specific statement, that such names are exempt from the relevant protective laws and regulations and therefore free for general use.
The publisher, the authors and the editors are safe to assume that the advice and information in this book are believed to be true and accurate at the date of publication. Neither the publisher nor the authors or the editors give a warranty, express or implied, with respect to the material contained herein or for any errors or omissions that may have been made. The publisher remains neutral with regard to jurisdictional claims in published maps and institutional affiliations.

Printed on acid-free paper

This Springer imprint is published by Springer Nature
The registered company is Springer International Publishing AG
The registered company address is: Gewerbestrasse 11, 6330 Cham, Switzerland

To my children, Annabel and Andrew, for their love and support, and my husband, Ken, for always being there for me and encouraging me.

A special gratitude to all my patients who serve as a powerful inspiration and allow me to share in their journey of courage and determination.

Antoinette R. Tan, MD, MHSc, FACP

Foreword

Triple-negative breast cancer as a relevant clinical entity did not exist until the routine incorporation of human epidermal growth factor receptor type 2 (HER2) testing along with hormone receptors in the late 1990s. Since that time, there has been an explosion of interest and research in this entity which remains to this day our most challenging clinical subset of breast cancer. From a risk standpoint, triple-negative breast cancer afflicts young women and women of color. From a treatment standpoint, it is the only subset of breast cancer for which we have no known targeted therapies. From a prognostic standpoint despite advances in chemotherapy, it remains the subset with poorest survival.

There is hope on the horizon. As genomic techniques have improved, it has become increasingly clear that triple-negative breast cancer is molecularly heterogeneous in ways that may be therapeutically relevant and identifiable. Chemotherapy regimens are increasingly tailored to appropriate clinical and risk strata. Novel approaches such as immune checkpoint inhibition, poly(ADP-ribose) polymerase (PARP) inhibition, and targeting alternative signaling pathways show promise. Someday "triple-negative breast cancer," which is defined by what it isn't, will be refined into treatable entities.

Triple-Negative Breast Cancer: A Clinician's Guide is designed for practicing clinicians. It is filled with clinical pearls as well as the new knowledge that is emerging to inform future practice. This guide reflects the multidisciplinary care that is optimal for these patients and is intended to foster effective understanding and communication, which are key to improved outcomes.

September 15, 2017   Lisa A. Carey, MD
                                    L. Richardson and Marilyn Jacobs Preyer
                            Distinguished Professor of Breast Cancer Research
                                                          Chapel Hill, NC
                                                                    USA

Preface

As a breast medical oncologist practicing in a hybrid academic-community cancer center system, I often receive questions on how I would manage a particular patient with triple-negative breast cancer or what would be my next treatment regimen in the setting of metastatic triple-negative disease. I felt that a practical handbook that could assist clinicians in managing triple-negative breast cancer patients in clinic could fill a special need.

This guide is designed for the practicing oncologist, fellow in training, and other healthcare professionals who are looking for a summary of the current thinking on the diagnosis, treatment, and management of triple-negative breast cancer. The content is in the form of review articles. Each chapter includes clinical pearls, or key messages, to assist providers in the multidisciplinary management of this disease.

This important handbook covers the pathologic evaluation, clinical features, genetics, imaging, and surgical management of triple-negative breast cancer. There are also evidence-based reviews of the different treatment modalities used to treat this disease, including radiation therapy, adjuvant therapy, and neoadjuvant chemotherapy for early-stage disease and chemotherapy treatment for metastatic disease. A look to ongoing developments in molecular profiling and emerging new data on targeted therapy is included. The specific issues that face both young women and elderly with triple-negative breast cancer are highlighted.

I would like to sincerely thank all the authors who are leaders in this field for donating their time and expertise to create this valuable tool. It is my hope that this book will help guide clinicians in their daily real-world practice of managing and treating patients with triple-negative breast cancer.

Charlotte, NC, USA   Antoinette R. Tan, MD, MHSc, FACP

Acknowledgments

Dr. Mootz and Dr. Dogan would like to thank Susannie Washington for her assistance in manuscript editing of their chapter.

.

Contents

1   Pathologic Evaluation of Triple-Negative Breast Cancer   1
    Chad A. Livasy

2   Triple-Negative Breast Cancer: Clinical Features   23
    Tira Tan and Rebecca Dent

3   The Genetics of Triple-Negative Breast Cancer   33
    Nanna H. Sulai and Olufunmilayo I. Olopade

4   Imaging of Triple-Negative Breast Cancer   41
    Ann R. Mootz and Basak E. Dogan

5   Surgical Management of Triple-Negative Breast Cancer   55
    Ali Amro and Lisa A. Newman

6   Radiation Therapy for Triple-Negative Breast Cancer   71
    Suzanne B. Evans and Bruce G. Haffty

7   Optimizing Adjuvant and Neoadjuvant Chemotherapy
    for Triple-Negative Breast Cancer   83
    Sonya Reid-Lawrence, Antoinette R. Tan, and Ingrid A. Mayer

8   Management of Metastatic Triple-Negative Breast Cancer   95
    Anne P. O'Dea and Priyanka Sharma

9   Molecular Profiling and Targeted Therapy
    for Triple-Negative Breast Cancer   117
    April T. Swoboda and Rita Nanda

10 Special Issues in Young Women with Triple-Negative
    Breast Cancer   141
    Narjust Duma, Ciara C. O'Sullivan, Kathryn J. Ruddy,
    and Alexis D. Leal

11 Individualizing the Approach to the Older Woman
    with Triple-Negative Breast Cancer   159
    Jasmeet Chadha Singh and Stuart M. Lichtman

Contributors

Ali Amro, MD Henry Ford Health System, Detroit, MI, USA

Rebecca Dent, MD, FRCP Division of Medical Oncology, National Cancer Centre Singapore, Singapore, Singapore

Basak E. Dogan, MD, FSBI Department of Diagnostic Radiology, The University of Texas Southwestern Medical Center, Dallas, TX, USA

Narjust Duma, MD Department of Oncology, Mayo Clinic College of Medicine and Science, Mayo Clinic, Rochester, MN, USA

Suzanne B. Evans, MD, MPH Department of Therapeutic Radiology, Yale University School of Medicine, New Haven, CT, USA

Bruce G. Haffty, MD, FASTRO Department of Radiation Oncology, Rutgers Cancer Institute of New Jersey, Rutgers Robert Wood Johnson Medical School, New Brunswick, NJ, USA

Alexis D. Leal, MD Division of Medical Oncology, University of Colorado Cancer Center, Aurora, CO, USA

Stuart M. Lichtman, MD Weill Cornell Medical College, Memorial Sloan Kettering Cancer Center, New York, NY, USA

Chad A. Livasy, MD Department of Pathology, Carolinas HealthCare System, Charlotte, NC, USA

Department of Pathology and Laboratory Medicine, University of North Carolina at Chapel Hill, Chapel Hill, NC, USA

Ingrid A. Mayer, MD, MSCI Division of Hematology/Oncology, Vanderbilt University Medical Center, Vanderbilt-Ingram Cancer Center, Nashville, TN, USA

Ann R. Mootz, MD Department of Diagnostic Radiology, The University of Texas Southwestern Medical Center, Dallas, TX, USA

Rita Nanda, MD Section of Hematology/Oncology, The University of Chicago Medicine, Chicago, IL, USA

Lisa A. Newman, MD, MPH, FACS, FASCO Henry Ford Cancer Institute, Detroit, MI, USA

Anne P. O'Dea, MD University of Kansas Medical Center, Westwood, KS, USA

Olufunmilayo I. Olopade, MD, FACP Department of Internal Medicine, Division of Hematology Oncology, University of Chicago Medical Center, Chicago, IL, USA

Ciara C. O'Sullivan, MB, BCh Department of Oncology, Mayo Clinic College of Medicine and Science, Mayo Clinic, Rochester, MN, USA

Sonya Reid-Lawrence, MBBS Division of Hematology/Oncology, Vanderbilt University Medical Center, Vanderbilt-Ingram Cancer Center, Nashville, TN, USA

Kathryn J. Ruddy, MD, MPH Department of Oncology, Mayo Clinic College of Medicine and Science, Mayo Clinic, Rochester, MN, USA

Priyanka Sharma, MD University of Kansas Medical Center, Westwood, KS, USA

Jasmeet Chadha Singh, MD Breast Medicine Division, Department of Medicine, Memorial Sloan Kettering Cancer Center, West Harrison, NY, USA

Nanna H. Sulai, MD Department of Solid Tumor Oncology and Investigational Therapeutics, Levine Cancer Institute, Carolinas HealthCare System, Charlotte, NC, USA

April T. Swoboda, MD Section of Hematology/Oncology, The University of Chicago Medicine, Chicago, IL, USA

Antoinette R. Tan, MD, MHSc, FACP Department of Solid Tumor Oncology and Investigational Therapeutics, Levine Cancer Institute, Carolinas HealthCare System, Charlotte, NC, USA

Tira Tan, BSc, MBBS, MRCP Division of Medical Oncology, National Cancer Centre Singapore, Singapore, Singapore

Pathologic Evaluation of Triple-Negative Breast Cancer

Chad A. Livasy

Clinical Pearls
- Accurate assessment of hormone receptor and human epidermal growth factor receptor type 2 status is critical to appropriately classify tumors into the triple-negative group.
- Triple-negative breast cancers (TNBCs) show significant morphologic and molecular heterogeneity.
- While the majority of TNBCs are ductal (no special type) tumors with aggressive natural history, rare histologic subtypes are associated with favorable prognosis, such as adenoid cystic carcinoma.
- Histologic features associated with triple-negative status include Nottingham grade 3 histology with high mitotic rate, pushing margin of invasion, geographic necrosis, lymphocytic infiltrate, large central acellular zone, metaplastic features, salivary gland differentiation, and apocrine differentiation.
- Other neoplasms involving the breast such as sarcoma, lymphoma, melanoma, and metastatic carcinoma from non-mammary primary may closely mimic TNBC.

1.1 Background

Systematic assessment of estrogen receptor (ER), progesterone receptor (PR), and human epidermal growth factor receptor 2 (HER2) status for invasive mammary carcinoma is the cornerstone of current clinical management of breast cancer as

C.A. Livasy, MD
Department of Pathology, Carolinas HealthCare System, Charlotte, NC, USA

Department of Pathology and Laboratory Medicine, University of North Carolina
at Chapel Hill, Chapel Hill, NC, USA
e-mail: chad.livasy@carolinashealthcare.org

© Springer International Publishing AG 2018
A.R. Tan (ed.), *Triple-Negative Breast Cancer*,
https://doi.org/10.1007/978-3-319-69980-6_1

these biomarkers predict benefit from endocrine and HER2-targeted therapies. ER-negative, PR-negative, and HER2-negative, so-called triple-negative breast cancers (TNBCs), are a heterogeneous subgroup and comprise approximately 15–20% of breast cancers. As this subgroup of tumors currently lacks effective targeted therapy agents, the main utility in grouping the TNBCs together, particularly high-grade ductal (no special type) and metaplastic carcinomas, is to focus research on identifying the mechanisms of carcinogenesis for these tumors and to develop effective novel therapies through clinical trials. Studies to date have highlighted the molecular diversity of TNBCs and the need for clinical trial design that takes this heterogeneity into consideration.

Several studies have shown inferior prognosis associated with triple-negative and basal-like breast cancers, particularly when compared to hormone receptor-positive tumors [1–6]. TNBCs have been shown to have an increased likelihood of distant recurrence and death within 5 years of diagnosis. Dent et al. studied 1601 patients with breast cancer and found that the risk of distant recurrence in TNBCs peaked around 3 years and declined rapidly thereafter [5]. In contrast, hormone receptor-positive tumors showed a recurrence risk that seemed to be constant over the period of follow-up. Other observations from their study of triple-negative tumors include a weak relationship between tumor size and node status, distant recurrence rarely preceded by local recurrence, local recurrence not predictive of distant recurrence, and rapid progression from distant recurrence to death.

Studies have shown uniqueness to the patterns of metastasis and relapse for TNBCs [5, 7]. Triple-negative tumors consistently show more aggressive visceral disease (e.g., lung) and soft tissue disease and less common bone relapse, when compared to hormone receptor-positive tumors. Triple-negative tumors have also been shown to be overrepresented in patients with brain metastasis. In one study of over 3000 patients, triple-negative status was the greatest risk factor for the development of cerebral metastasis [8].

The TNBCs are a heterogeneous group of tumors and include rare histologic subtypes showing a more favorable prognosis. Clinicians may be unaware of the more favorable prognosis associated with rare histologic subtypes of TNBC including adenoid cystic carcinoma, secretory carcinoma, low-grade adenosquamous carcinoma, and low-grade fibromatosis-like carcinoma (Table 1.1). For pathologists, it is important to clarify the prognostic significance of these rare histologic subtypes in the pathology report, emphasizing the continued need to interpret triple-negative status in the context of tumor grade and histology.

Table 1.1 Triple-negative breast cancer rare histologic subtypes associated with favorable prognosis

Adenoid cystic carcinoma
Secretory carcinoma
Low-grade adenosquamous carcinoma
Low-grade fibromatosis-like carcinoma

1.2 Pathologic Assessment of Breast Cancer Receptor Status

The classification of an invasive mammary carcinoma as triple-negative is based on pathologic evaluation of the tumor for ER, PR, and HER2 expression (Table 1.2). Immunohistochemistry (IHC) is the accepted methodology for evaluation of ER and PR expression. IHC and in situ hybridization (ISH) are both acceptable methodologies for evaluating HER2 status. It is premature to recommend alternative methodologies such as mRNA by reverse transcription polymerase chain reaction (RT-PCR) or DNA microarray assays in unselected patients. The current guidelines recommend that ER and PR assays be resulted as positive if there are at least 1% positive tumor nuclei in the sample on testing in the presence of expected reactivity of internal and external controls [9]. If less than 1% of tumor cell nuclei are immunoreactive for ER and PR, the sample is considered hormone receptor-negative based on data that such patients do not receive meaningful benefit from endocrine therapy. Testing criteria define HER2-negative if a single test (or all tests) performed on tumor specimen shows (a) IHC 1+ negative or IHC 0 negative or (b) ISH negative using single-probe (average HER2 copy <4 signals/cell) or dual-probe ISH negative (HER2/CEP17 ratio <2.0 with an average HER2 copy number <4.0 signals/cells) [10].

Accurate testing is essential in appropriately classifying the tumor receptor status and guiding therapy. Pre-analytic, analytic, and post-analytic variables may all affect the quality of receptor testing results and must be controlled to ensure that the assay results reflect the true receptor status of the tumor. In an effort to improve the accuracy of receptor testing and the utility of ER, PR, and HER2 as prognostic and predictive markers for invasive breast carcinoma, multiple guideline recommendations for ER, PR, and HER2 testing have been issued by international expert panels convened by the ASCO and the CAP [9, 10]. It is important that clinicians are aware of some key components of these recommendations to help ensure accurate testing and interpretation of results.

Table 1.2 Criteria for classifying invasive breast cancer as triple-negative

Receptor	Result
Estrogen receptor IHC	<1% of tumor cell nuclei staining (of any intensity) in presence of adequate controls
Progesterone receptor IHC	<1% of tumor cell nuclei staining (of any intensity) in presence of adequate controls
HER2 IHC or ISH	One or both tests showing:
	IHC
	• Score 0 or 1+
	ISH
	• Single-probe average HER2 copy number <4.0 signals/cell
	• Dual-probe HER2/CEP17 <2.0 with average of <4.0 HER2 signals/cell

Important pre-analytic variables that may affect receptor results include cold ischemic time (time from excision of tissue to initiation of fixation), type of fixative, volume of fixative in relation to volume of tissue, and duration of fixation. The guideline recommendation in regard to pre-analytic variables states that breast specimens must be fixed in an adequate volume of 10% neutral-buffered formalin for no less than 6 h and for no longer than 72 h before processing. Additionally, the cold ischemic time should be kept to ≤1 h. The breast care management team needs to be aware of these guidelines to help ensure that procedures are in place to track both cold ischemic time and duration of fixation. In regard to cold ischemic time, it is important that formalin be in direct contact with the tumor to optimize fixation. Tissue treatment of bone biopsies with decalcifying agents may also affect receptor expression levels leading to false negative result or preclude hybridization leading to no result for ISH studies. A cautionary statement in the pathology report should be added to negative receptor interpretations for specimens treated with decalcifying agents, particularly when the result is discordant with the breast primary.

In certain circumstances, retesting of ER/PR and/or HER2 may be indicated before classifying a tumor as hormone receptor-negative or HER2-negative. If the receptor findings are discordant with tumor histology, such as hormone receptor-negative or HER2-positive results for a Nottingham grade 1 tubular, lobular, cribriform, or mucinous carcinoma (which are almost always hormone receptor-positive and HER2-negative), repeat testing should be considered. If the initial core biopsy is HER2-negative and the excision specimen contains high-grade carcinoma that is morphologically distinct from the core biopsy, repeat HER2 testing is indicated on the resection specimen, as these findings may be indicative of intratumoral HER2 genetic heterogeneity. Retesting of an alternative specimen should be performed, if possible, when there is doubt about the specimen handling (e.g., long cold ischemic time, short or extended time in fixative, alternative fixative) or unexpected results following specimen decalcification.

The introduction of an equivocal category for HER2 testing by ISH may complicate the classification of tumors in regard to triple-negative status, particularly for hormone receptor-negative, HER2 double equivocal (by both IHC and ISH) tumors. It should be noted that tumors with final ISH findings that fall into the current equivocal definition (HER2/CEP17 ratio <2.0 and average HER2 copy number ≥4.0 and <6.0 signals per cell) were classified as HER2-negative in the first-generation trastuzumab clinical trials. There is lack of data on the response to HER2-targeted therapy in the subgroup of patients with HER2 equivocal results. Data from the National Surgical Adjuvant Breast and Bowel Project (NSABP) B-47 trial may help determine the value of adjuvant HER2-targeted therapies in patients whose breast cancers show low levels of HER2 expression.

Prior to standardization of criteria to classify tumors as hormone receptor-positive, many investigators and clinicians considered 10% or greater nuclear staining as the threshold for defining hormone receptor-positive status and therefore eligibility for endocrine therapy. Gene expression profiling studies of tumors showing low hormone receptor-positive status (1–9% nuclei staining) frequently show basal-like molecular characteristics for these tumors and a minority with luminal B features [11]. While the ASCO/CAP panel recommends considering endocrine therapy in patients whose tumors show 1–9% weakly positive cells, there is recognition that it is reasonable for oncologists to discuss the pros and cons of endocrine therapy with patients whose tumors express low levels of ER and make an informed decision based on the balance.

1.3   Gene Expression Profiling Studies

Gene expression profiling of breast cancers has identified unique biologic subtypes associated with survival outcomes and resulted in new classification schemes [1–3]. Not only can TNBCs be classified into several "intrinsic" molecular subtypes (luminal A/luminal B, basal-like, HER2-enriched, and claudin-low) but also into six transcriptomic subtypes with potential therapeutic implications (basal-like 1, basal-like 2, immunomodulatory, luminal androgen receptor, mesenchymal-like, and mesenchymal stem-like) [12]. The clinical value of these molecular classification systems for TNBCs will need to be determined by prospective validation in clinical trials.

The seminal work by Perou, Sorlie, and colleagues identified a subtype of breast cancer termed basal-like due to its similarity to the expression pattern observed in normal breast basal/myoepithelial cells [1]. While most TNBCs cluster with basal-like or claudin-low subtypes (approximately 80%), TNBCs are observed within each of the intrinsic subtypes identified by gene expression profiling [12, 13]. Basal-like carcinomas show expression of basal cytokeratins 5 and 17, EGFR, and proliferation genes (including Ki-67 and PCNA) and downregulation of ER, PR, and HER2 expression [14–18]. This group is homogeneously highly proliferative contributing to the rapid growth observed in these tumors. These tumors show high rates of *TP53* pathway alterations (frequent *TP53* mutation), frequent germline or somatic *BRCA* mutations (BRCAness), high rates of *RB* pathway alteration, high genomic instability, and hypomethylation compared with other breast cancer subtypes [19].

The rarer claudin-low subtype is commonly triple-negative and characterized by low to absent expression of luminal differentiation markers, high enrichment for epithelial-to-mesenchymal transition (EMT) markers, expression of immune response genes, and cancer stem cell-like features [20]. This cancer subtype is frequently seen in breast cancers with metaplastic differentiation.

The most common early genetic event in TNBC is a mutation of *TP53*, seen in approximately 80–85% of cases [21, 22]. A wide variety of less common genetic events have been identified highlighting the molecular diversity observed in TNBCs. These genetic abnormalities include *MYC* amplification (40%), *MCL1* amplification (20%), *RB1* mutation or loss (20%), sporadic/germline *BRCA* 1 or 2 mutation (15–20%), *PTEN* mutation/deletion (10%), *CCNE1* amplification (9%) and *USH2A* mutation (9%), *PIK3CA* mutation (8%), *FGFR2* amplification (4%), and *HER2* mutation (2%) [21–24].

Fig. 1.1 Triple-negative breast cancer commonly demonstrates a circumscribed and lobulated border. The cut surfaces are typically tan and firm and may demonstrate foci of yellow necrosis as seen in the central aspects of this tumor

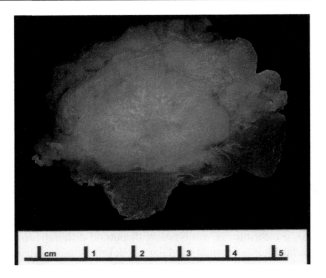

1.4   Gross Features

TNBCs show a wide range of variation in their gross appearance. TNBCs are less likely to demonstrate spiculated margins and associated calcifications, as compared to non-TNBCs. These tumors have an increased propensity to show a more circumscribed gross appearance when compared to hormone receptor-positive tumors (Fig. 1.1). When these well-circumscribed spherical tumors present in young women, they can be confused with fibroadenoma on physical exam and imaging studies. Rarely, TNBC may present as a cystic or cystic and solid mass. Due in large part to the high proliferative rate of most of these tumors, the average presenting tumor size for triple-negative tumors is larger than that observed for hormone receptor-positive tumors. The cut surface of these tumors ranges from tan to gray/white and may show varying degrees of necrosis. The necrotic foci often appear yellow or red/brown when associated with hemorrhage. Some variants show extensive central necrosis or a large central fibrotic zone.

1.5   Histopathology No Special Type (Ductal) Triple-Negative Breast Cancer

TNBCs show tremendous diversity in their histopathologic appearance (Table 1.3). The vast majority of TNBCs are ductal (no special type) carcinomas, and many of these tumors show some overlapping histopathologic features (Fig. 1.2). Microscopic features most frequently observed in ductal (no special type) carcinomas with a triple-negative phenotype include Nottingham grade 3 histology with high mitotic rate, pushing margin of invasion, lymphoid stroma, and geographic necrosis [25]. Not surprisingly, many of these histopathologic features overlap with

Table 1.3 Histologic features associated with triple-negative phenotype

• Grade 3 histology with high mitotic rate
• Pushing margin of invasion
• Geographic tumor necrosis
• Lymphocytic stromal response
• Solid-/sheetlike or ribbon-like growth patterns
• Large central zone of fibrosis/necrosis
• Metaplastic differentiation
• Myoepithelial differentiation
• Salivary gland differentiation
• Apocrine differentiation
• Secretory differentiation

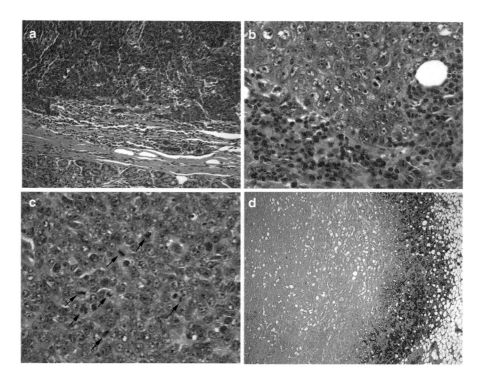

Fig. 1.2 Low-power magnification demonstrates solid sheetlike architecture with pushing margin of invasion, typical of a ductal (no special type) triple-negative breast cancer (**a**). Higher magnification demonstrates stromal tumor-infiltrating lymphocytes (TILs) at the peripheral edge of invasive carcinoma with high-grade nuclei (**b**) and markedly elevated mitotic index (mitotic figures indicated by arrows) (**c**). Large central acellular fibrotic focus surrounded by rim of viable high-grade invasive carcinoma (**d**)

those described as associated with invasive basal-like breast cancers. Histologic features of basal-like breast cancers identified by gene microarray analysis include markedly elevated mitotic rate ($P < 0.0001$), geographic tumor necrosis ($P < 0.0001$), pushing margin of invasion ($P = 0.0001$), and lymphocytic response

($P = 0.01$) [16]. Many triple-negative ductal carcinomas also show tumor cells with high nuclear/cytoplasmic ratios, solid-/sheetlike architecture pattern, and a syncytial arrangement of tumor cells. The constellation of findings in several of these tumors containing a prominent lymphoplasmacytic stromal infiltrate is similar to those previously used to describe medullary and atypical medullary carcinomas [26]. Rarely TNBCs may demonstrate marked nuclear pleomorphism with associated multinucleation.

Other less common ductal architectural patterns associated with triple-negative status include large, central fibrotic acellular zone and ribbon-like architecture associated with central necrosis (Fig. 1.2). Tsuda et al. described a series of high-grade invasive ductal carcinomas with large, central acellular zones showing aggressive clinical behavior and myoepithelial differentiation [27, 28]. In our experience, tumors with this morphology frequently show a triple-negative phenotype.

The vast majority of invasive breast cancers associated with germline *BRCA1* mutation show ductal (no special type) histology with a triple-negative phenotype and a basal-like subtype by gene expression profiling [29–32]. *BRCA1*-associated breast cancers frequently show a common constellation of histopathologic features including tumor circumscription, sheetlike growth pattern, lymphoid infiltrate, high mitotic rate, prominent nucleoli, and necrosis [33]. These observations indicate that the morphology and receptor status of a breast cancer can assist in the triaging of patients for genetic testing. Attention to the histologic features of a patient's breast cancer can improve selection criteria for genetic testing, thus improving sensitivity to detect *BRCA1* mutations. Farshid et al. demonstrated that morphology could predict the likelihood of association with a *BRCA1* mutation in a series of breast cancers with a sensitivity of 92%, specificity of 86%, positive predictive value of 61%, and negative predictive value of 98% [33].

1.6   Metaplastic Carcinoma

Metaplastic carcinomas show marked diversity in their histopathologic features and are almost exclusively triple-negative. These unusual tumors comprise approximately 1% of all breast cancers and usually demonstrate high-grade histology. By definition, these tumors demonstrate metaplastic differentiation of neoplastic epithelium into squamous cells and/or mesenchymal elements such as spindled/sarcomatoid, chondroid, osseous, and/or rhabdomyoid cells (Fig. 1.3). These tumors may be both entirely composed of metaplastic elements or a complex admixture of conventional ductal carcinoma and metaplastic areas.

High-grade invasive metaplastic carcinomas appear to have some unique clinical features including inherently aggressive tumor biology. Studies suggest that as a group metaplastic carcinomas have lower response rates to conventional adjuvant chemotherapy and worse clinical outcomes than those with other forms of TNBC. Jung et al. studied outcomes of 45 metaplastic breast carcinomas as compared to 473 triple-negative invasive ductal carcinomas [34]. Metaplastic histology

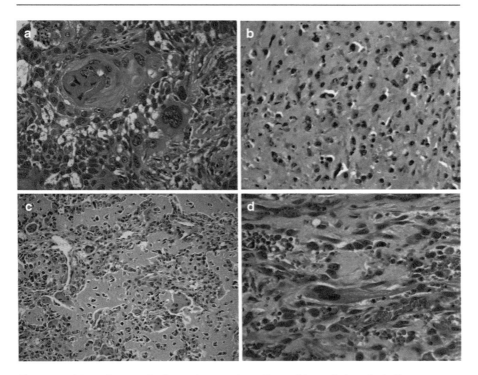

Fig. 1.3 High-grade metaplastic carcinomas show diverse histopathology including squamous differentiation with keratin pearl formation (**a**), chondroid matrix formation (**b**), osteoid matrix formation (**c**), and high-grade sarcomatous differentiation (**d**)

was a poor prognostic factor for disease recurrence and overall survival in univariate and multivariate analysis. Poorer clinical outcomes were observed as compared to ductal (no special type) TNBC. Chen et al. examined a group of 11 patients with locally advanced T3–T4 metaplastic carcinoma who received neoadjuvant chemotherapy, and only two patients exhibited a partial response [35]. Lymph node metastases are significantly less frequently found in metaplastic carcinomas as compared to ductal (no special type) carcinomas, and hematogenous metastases preferentially affecting the lungs and brain are more likely. By gene expression profiling, most metaplastic carcinomas are classified as either claudin-low/mesenchymal-like or basal-like. Whole exome sequencing studies of metaplastic carcinoma show that these tumors are complex and heterogeneous with more frequent mutations in PI3K/AKT/mTOR and Wnt pathways, as compared to ductal (no special type) TNBCs [36].

It should be noted that there are exceptionally rare forms of triple-negative metaplastic carcinoma that limited studies have indicated are associated with a more favorable prognosis. These more favorable subtypes are low-grade adenosquamous carcinoma (LG-ASC) and low-grade fibromatosis-like carcinoma

(LG-FLC). LG-ASC demonstrates infiltrative low-grade glandular and tubular structures and solid nests of squamous cells in a spindle cell background. LG-ASC may be seen arising in association with papilloma, radial scar, or sclerosing adenosis. Lymph node involvement by LG-ASC is extremely rare, with only one documented case [37]. Similarly, there is only one documented case of systemic disease due to LG-ASC in a patient who presented with an 8.0 cm breast mass and lung metastases [37]. LG-ASC may recur locally if incompletely excised. Low-grade fibromatosis-like carcinoma is comprised of infiltrative cytologically bland spindle cells that mimic fibromatosis or other spindle cell lesions of the breast; however, most of these tumors show as least focal cytokeratin expression by immunohistochemistry. Although risk of regional lymph node involvement is low, 0 of 15 patients in one study where patients underwent axillary lymph node dissection, rarely these tumors may demonstrate hematogenous metastases to the lungs [38, 39]. LG-FLC may be locally aggressive. One study demonstrated a high local recurrence rate of 44% (8 of 18 patients), recurring up to 88 months after initial surgery [39].

1.7   Apocrine Carcinoma

Apocrine carcinomas are rare tumors, comprising <1% of invasive breast cancers when strict criteria for diagnosis are applied. Overall, most patients with apocrine carcinoma tend to be postmenopausal and about 5–10 years older than patients with non-apocrine ductal carcinomas [40]. The designation of apocrine carcinoma should be reserved for tumors in which all or nearly all of the epithelium has apocrine morphology. Focal apocrine differentiation may be observed in many histologic subtypes of invasive breast cancer. Apocrine cytology is characterized by cells with abundant cytoplasm that is densely eosinophilic and granular and large nuclei containing vesicular chromatin and prominent nucleoli (Fig. 1.4a). Tumors showing prominent apocrine differentiation are almost always hormone receptor-negative, but not necessarily triple-negative. A significant subset of these tumors, approximately 30–50%, will show HER2 overexpression, with the remainder being triple-negative [41]. The majority of these tumors show increased androgen receptor (AR) expression and strong positive staining for gross cystic disease fluid protein 15 (GCDFP-15), a marker of apocrine differentiation [42]. As a group these tumors exhibit a lower proliferative rate as compared to ductal (no special type) TNBCs [43]. Outcome studies have shown no statistically significant differences between apocrine carcinoma and non-apocrine carcinomas in recurrence-free survival or overall survival [44]. Although studies are limited, Nagao et al. evaluated five patients with invasive apocrine carcinoma who underwent neoadjuvant chemotherapy and experienced only minimal reduction in size, and no pathologic complete responses were observed [45].

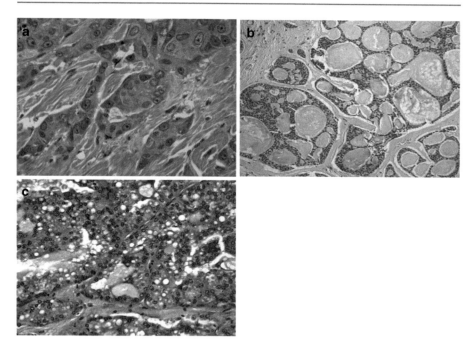

Fig. 1.4 Apocrine carcinomas contain tumor cells with abundant eosinophilic granular cytoplasm and large nuclei containing vesicular chromatin and prominent nucleoli (**a**). Adenoid cystic carcinoma with cribriform pattern comprised of pseudolumina containing myxoid spherules of basement membrane material that are surrounded by small basaloid cells with low nuclear grade (**b**). The very rare secretory carcinoma demonstrates prominent cytoplasmic secretory vacuoles and low-grade nuclear features (**c**)

1.8   Adenoid Cystic Carcinoma

Adenoid cystic carcinoma (ACC) is a rare special type of TNBC comprising <0.1% of breast carcinomas and is associated with a particularly favorable prognosis [46]. The reported 10-year survival rate for patients with mammary ACC is >90% [46–48]. Most of the deaths reported from mammary ACC are due to tumors with histologic features that deviated from the classic histopathologic definition. Mammary ACC shows indolent biologic behavior and extremely low capacity for regional lymph node involvement.

Microscopic evaluation of ACC shows an admixture of epithelial (luminal) and myoepithelial (basal) cell types often arranged into classic tubular and cribriform patterns (Fig. 1.4b). The neoplastic cells are polarized around two types of structures: true glandular spaces and pseudolumina. The true glandular spaces contain neutral periodic acid-Schiff (PAS)-positive mucin and are surrounded by cytokeratin 7-positive luminal epithelial cells that tend to have more abundant cytoplasm than the admixed basal/myoepithelial cells. The epithelial component can assume variable architectural patterns including solid, cribriform, tubular, and trabecular configurations. Pseudolumina result from intraluminal invaginations of stroma containing myxoid material or eosinophilic spherules of basement membrane components. The pseudolumina are of varying shape, mostly round, and are surrounded by basal/myoepithelial cells that typically show positive staining for a variety of myoepithelial/basal markers including p63, smooth muscle myosin heavy chain, calponin, and basal cytokeratins (cytokeratin 5/6, cytokeratin 14, cytokeratin 17). The nuclear features of the luminal epithelial and basal/myoepithelial cells are low grade and the mitotic rate is low. Foci of cellular necrosis are typically absent. In contrast to salivary gland ACC, perineural invasion is usually not observed.

A grading system specific for mammary ACC has been proposed and is based on the proportion of solid growth observed within the tumor [49]. This grading system divides ACC into three groups (grade 1, no solid elements; grade 2, <30% solid pattern; grade 3, ≥30% solid pattern). This single study reported that grade 2 and 3 tumors have a tendency to be larger and were more likely to develop recurrences. The prognostic utility of this grading system has not been confirmed by other studies [50]. The American Joint Committee on Cancer Staging Manual recommends that Nottingham histologic grading be provided for all breast carcinomas. Based on this grading scheme, most ACCs would be graded as Nottingham grade 1 or 2.

One particularly rare histologic variant of ACC has been termed solid variant of mammary ACC with basaloid features [51]. These tumors are characterized by nearly (>90%) or entirely solid growth pattern with basaloid appearance of tumor cells. In contrast to conventional ACC, these tumors may also show moderate to marked nuclear atypia, brisk mitotic activity, and loss of demonstrable myoepithelial differentiation. It is controversial whether all of these tumors truly represent a form of ACC or are part of the spectrum of basaloid ductal (no special type) carcinomas. For tumors that show histologic features that depart from the classically described ACC, particularly those showing loss of demonstrable myoepithelial differentiation, assurance of indolent biologic behavior is lost. Molecular studies have not been shown to resolve the classification of these rare variant tumors.

ACCs, regardless of site of origin, harbor the recurrent t (6; 9) (q22–23; p23–24) translocation that results in the formation of the *MYB-NFIB* fusion gene [52, 53]. This results in activation and overexpression of *MYB* at the mRNA and protein levels. *MYB* is a leucine zipper transcription factor that plays an important role in the control of cell proliferation, apoptosis, and differentiation. Although a portion of ACCs lack the *MYB-NFIB* fusion gene, these tumors are likely to display activation of *MYB* due to mechanisms other than the t (6; 9) chromosomal translocation [54]. Although the *MYB-NFIB* fusion gene is a characteristic of mammary ACC, the diagnosis ACC in breast biopsies is still based on the characteristic histopathologic and immunophenotypic features of this rare tumor type.

Detailed molecular studies of mammary ACCs have demonstrated a low exonic mutation rate, low levels of genetic instability, and a heterogeneous constellation of somatic genetic alterations targeting chromatin remodeling, cell adhesion, and canonical signaling pathway genes, including mutations in cancer genes such as *BRAF*, *FBXW7*, *FGFR2*, and *MTOR* [55–57]. The mutations and copy number variations seen in common triple-negative and basal-like ductal carcinomas, such as mutations in p53 and 4p, 5q, and 10q losses and 6p, 8q, and 10p gains, are not typically found in mammary ACC [55, 58, 59]. Aneuploidy is reported in less than 10% of breast ACCs [60]. Studies have demonstrated significantly higher levels of *BRCA1* mRNA in ACCs than in the common types of triple-negative or basal-like breast cancers, indicating retention of normal *BRCA1* function [55]. Altogether, these molecular studies demonstrate that mammary ACCs are a distinct form of triple-negative breast carcinoma sharing a genomic landscape much more similar to salivary gland ACCs than to the more common forms of triple-negative or basal-like breast carcinomas.

1.9   Secretory Carcinoma

Secretory carcinomas are a very rare translocation-associated invasive carcinoma characterized by marked secretory changes including eosinophilic vacuolated cytoplasm and prominent intra- and extracellular eosinophilic secretions, usually located within the lumen of tubules (Fig. 1.4c). Clinically, these tumors often present as circumscribed masses and may present in children, with reported age ranging from 3 to 91 years [61–63]. Gross exam of these tumors typically shows a circumscribed, firm mass which may be lobulated. Histologically, most tumors show a combination of microcystic, solid, and tubular architecture and a pushing border of invasion. Mitotic activity is minimal within these tumors. Secretory carcinomas show variable receptor findings, but the majority of these tumors demonstrate a triple-negative phenotype. Secretory carcinoma is associated with a characteristic balanced translocation, t(12;15), that creates an *ETV6-NTRK3* gene fusion [64]. STAT5a, a mammary growth factor, is often positive in secretory carcinoma. Activity of this growth factor may explain the secretory properties of the tumor cells. Activation of STAT5a in the breast typically occurs as a result of prolactin binding to its receptor. It has been postulated that in secretory carcinoma, unregulated kinase activity of the fusion gene leads to phosphorylation of STAT5a and activation of its downstream pathways [65]. Secretory carcinomas follow a low-grade clinical course resulting in an exceptionally favorable prognosis. Local recurrence and regional lymph node metastases have been reported [66–70]. Distant metastases and death from secretory carcinoma are extremely rare, limited to case reports [69, 71, 72].

1.10   Pathologic Differential Diagnosis

The diagnosis of most TNBCs is typically straightforward. Due to the lack of differentiation in many of these tumors, including absence of tubule formation, the differential diagnosis in biopsy specimens includes large cell lymphoma, sarcoma (particularly angiosarcoma), metastatic carcinoma from non-mammary primary, and metastatic malignant melanoma. Histologically, these other tumors may closely mimic a TNBC. Difficulty in excluding these other neoplasms on morphology alone is exaggerated on core biopsies where there is limited sampling of the tumor. It is important that clinical history of any other malignancy is clearly communicated on the surgical pathology requisition to alert the pathologist to potential metastasis from a non-mammary site. Advanced stage carcinoma from a wide variety of sites, including lung, gastrointestinal tract, or gynecologic tract, may metastasize to the breast and mimic a breast primary. Metastatic carcinoma to the breast should be considered in any patient with history of non-mammary carcinoma and new breast lesion. Metastatic tumors are rarely spiculated on imaging studies and often present as a rounded nodule or density, and multiple lesions may be present. Special immunohistochemical stains are able to ascertain breast primary versus metastasis in the vast majority cases.

The diffuse solid growth pattern of large cell lymphoma may closely resemble some TNBCs, but the lymphocytes typically show less striking nuclear atypia with small to absent nucleoli and increased cellular discohesion compared to carcinomas. Immunohistochemical stains for pan-cytokeratin, CD20, and CD3 easily distinguish these entities.

Spindle cell metaplastic carcinomas, depending on nuclear grade, may show similar histopathologic features to malignant phyllodes tumor (high nuclear grade) or fibromatosis (low nuclear grade). The most likely diagnosis for every sarcomatous-appearing lesion in the breast is metaplastic carcinoma. Focal epithelioid features are present in the majority of high-grade sarcomatoid metaplastic carcinomas and a major clue to the correct diagnosis. A panel of high and low molecular weight cytokeratins is recommended in these lesions to evaluate for epithelial differentiation where positive staining is supportive of metaplastic carcinoma. Definitive classification of a high-grade malignant spindle cell lesion (metaplastic spindle cell carcinoma vs malignant phyllodes tumor) on core biopsy may not always be possible with classification deferred to the excision specimen. Similarly, distinction of metaplastic low-grade fibromatosis-like carcinoma from mammary fibromatosis may be particularly problematic. An immunohistochemical panel of broad-spectrum cytokeratins, p63, and β-catenin is recommended for these cases where keratin and p63 expression support the diagnosis of carcinoma, and absent keratin/p63 staining and nuclear β-catenin expression support the diagnosis of fibromatosis.

Primary breast sarcomas that may closely mimic TNBC include angiosarcoma and undifferentiated sarcoma. The clinical context is often helpful in raising suspicion for sarcoma. High-grade malignant neoplasms arising in the breast 5–10 years post breast radiation therapy should raise suspicion for possible sarcoma. Skin changes noted on physical exam may raise suspicion for angiosarcoma and, if present, can be communicated to the pathologist to raise suspicion for the diagnosis of angiosarcoma. Immunostain for the endothelial marker CD31 is particularly helpful in assessing for angiosarcoma. As angiosarcomas may show focal positive staining for cytokeratin, a panel of immunostains is often required to establish the diagnosis.

1.11   Tumor-Infiltrating Lymphocytes

TNBCs characteristically contain more mutations than other types of breast cancer and may induce an immune response due to the presence of neoantigens. There is mounting evidence that immune system influences prognosis for breast cancer. Lymphocytic infiltration associated with breast cancer was described decades ago, particularly in association with high-grade tumors [73]. Interest in tumor-infiltrating lymphocytes (TILs) has increased as recent studies have demonstrated that stromal lymphocytic infiltration is a robust prognostic factor for TNBC. TILs were evaluated in 506 TNBCs from two randomized phase III clinical trials, ECOG 2197 and ECOG 1199, of adjuvant anthracycline-containing chemotherapy [74]. At a median follow-up of 10.6 years, higher stromal TIL scores were associated with better prognosis: for every 10% increase in lymphocytes, there was a risk reduction of 14% recurrence or death, 18% for distant recurrence, and 19% for death. Multivariate analysis confirmed stromal TILs to be an independent prognostic marker of disease-free survival, distant recurrence-free interval, and overall survival for TNBC. For TNBCs, the more stromal TILs a patient has at diagnosis, the better their outcome after adjuvant anthracycline-based chemotherapy. Although quantitation of stromal TILs is not yet part of routine pathology synoptic reporting, methods for quantitation have been proposed. There is currently no universally accepted standardized system for diagnostic applications.

The International TILs Work Group has proposed a methodology for quantitation of TILs in breast cancer specimens [75]. These recommendations include reporting of stromal TIL percentage, defined as the percentage of tumor stroma containing lymphocytes. More specifically, TILs should be reported as the percentage of stromal compartment area at the border of the invasive tumors occupied by all mononuclear inflammatory cells including lymphocytes and plasma cells (i.e., stromal area occupied by TILs over total stromal area). TILs may be assessed on core biopsies as well as surgical excisions. Although definitions have varied among studies, most studies have used 50–60% stromal TIL threshold to define lymphocyte-predominant breast cancer. To date, functional analyses of the immune cell infiltrates have not been clearly shown to add additional prognostic information.

1.12   Immunohistochemistry

A tremendous number of studies have addressed the immunohistochemical profile of triple-negative and basal-like breast cancers. The definitions and nomenclature used in these studies are inconsistent and have led to confusion about classification of both triple-negative and basal-like breast cancers. In addition to lack of hormone receptor expression and HER2 overexpression/amplification, one of the main characteristics of basal-like carcinomas is that they express basal cytokeratins (e.g., cytokeratin 5 and cytokeratin 17) [15, 76, 77]. While the identification of basal cytokeratin expression in triple-negative tumors is confirmatory of a basal-like subtype, not all basal-like carcinomas demonstrate positivity for basal cytokeratins by immunohistochemistry. Surrogate immunohistochemical studies to define tumors as basal-like have used different criteria to define a tumor as basal-like and have demonstrated significant immunophenotypic heterogeneity among these tumors. The most widely used immunohistochemical surrogate to define a tumor as basal-like is that proposed by Nielsen et al., where basal-like carcinomas were defined as those lacking ER and HER2 expression and expressing cytokeratin 5/6 and/or EGFR [15]. This four-biomarker panel demonstrated a sensitivity of 76% and a specificity of 100%. There is currently no internationally accepted standard on biomarkers used to identify a tumor as basal-like, and the routine use of the term "basal-like" in pathology reports is not indicated. Many other biomarkers are reported to be associated with triple-negative and basal-like carcinoma and are listed in Table 1.4 [15, 18, 21, 22, 77–97]. Two of these biomarkers, androgen receptor (AR) and PD-L1, are discussed in greater detail below.

Some TNBCs appear to be driven by hormonal pathways involving androgens. Depending on the threshold used to define positive expression, AR is expressed in 10–75% of TNBCs [95–97]. By gene expression profiling, the luminal androgen receptor group is enriched in hormone-regulated pathways with high AR expression at both the mRNA and protein levels [12]. This group demonstrates a luminal gene expression signature and a low proliferative rate. Androgen-driven TNBCs have different response rates and survival outcomes compared with other TNBC subgroups. Histologically, several of these tumors demonstrate prominent apocrine differentiation. The utility of targeted AR inhibition therapy is being explored in clinical trials.

Table 1.4 Immunohistochemical biomarkers associated with triple-negative or basal-like carcinomas

• Basal cytokeratins (cytokeratins 5 and 17)
• Epidermal growth factor receptor (EGFR)
• Vimentin
• p53
• p63
• Androgen receptor (AR)
• p16
• Laminin
• Maspin
• Nestin
• Fascin
• P-cadherin
• Cyclin A, E and B1
• c-KIT
• Caveolin-1 and caveolin-2
• αβ-Crystallin
• Proliferation-associated proteins (Ki-67 and PCNA)
• ALDH1
• CD44
• PD-L1

There is increasing recognition that some breast cancers acquire the ability to evade the immune system. Tumor expression of programmed cell death ligand 1 (PD-L1) is associated with immune evasion and expressed in a subset of TNBCs [93, 94]. Studies to date have demonstrated PD-L1 expression in breast cancer is more prevalent among high-grade, hormone receptor-negative breast cancers with a range of histologic appearance. Dill et al. evaluated 245 primary breast cancers and found PD-L1 expression in 32% of TNBCs; however, diffuse (>50%) staining was rare (5% of TNBCs) [93]. Intratumoral heterogeneity in PD-L1 expression was observed. In cases with matched primary/metastatic pairs, tumor PD-L1 expression was conserved in 94% of cases. Currently, data showing a strong correlation between PD-L1 expression in breast cancer and response to immune checkpoint inhibitors is lacking.

Conclusion

TNBCs, defined by absence of clinically significant expression of ER, PR, and HER2, comprise approximately 15–20% of all invasive breast cancer diagnoses. Accurate pathologic assessment of tumor ER, PR, and HER2 status is a critical part of appropriately classifying tumors into this subset. Pre-analytic, analytic, and post-analytic variables may all affect the quality of receptor testing results and must be controlled to ensure that the assay results reflect the true receptor status of the tumor. The definition of TNBC has been standardized with the publication of national guidelines on ER, PR, and HER2 testing/reporting by the ASCO and CAP. TNBCs show tremendous morphologic diversity including multiple unique histologic subtypes. While most TNBCs are ductal (no special type) carcinomas associated with aggressive natural history, rare histologic subtypes of TNBC are associated with favorable prognosis and highlight the continued need to link histologic subtype with triple-negative status. Gene expression profile studies have demonstrated molecular heterogeneity of TNBC, including identification of basal-like and claudin-low/mesenchymal-like subtypes. Other studies of TNBC have identified biologic features in a subset of these tumors with potential therapeutic implications including inactivation of the *BRCA* pathway, increased tumor-infiltrating lymphocytes (TILs), detection of immune gene signatures including increased PD-L1 expression, and androgen receptor expression.

References

1. Perou CM, Sorlie T, Eisen MB, et al. Molecular portraits of human breast tumours. Nature. 2000;406:747–52.
2. Sorlie T, Perou C, Tibshirani R, et al. Gene expression patterns of breast carcinomas distinguish tumor subclasses with clinical implications. Proc Natl Acad Sci U S A. 2001;98:10869–74.
3. Sorlie T, Tibshirani R, Parker J, et al. Repeated observation of breast tumor subtypes in independent gene expression data sets. Proc Natl Acad Sci U S A. 2003;100:8418–23.
4. Carey L, Perou C, Livasy C, et al. Race, breast cancer subtypes, and survival in the Carolina breast cancer study. JAMA. 2006;295:2492–502.

5. Dent R, Trudeau M, Pritchard KI, Hanna WM, et al. Triple-negative breast cancer: clinical features and patterns of recurrence. Clin Cancer Res. 2007;13:4429–34.

6. Liedtke C, Mazouni C, Hess K, et al. Response to neoadjuvant therapy and long-term survival in patients with triple-negative breast cancer. J Clin Oncol. 2008;26:1275–81.

7. Smid M, Wang Y, Zhang Y, et al. Subtypes of breast cancer show preferential site of relapse. Cancer Res. 2008;68:3108–14.

8. Heitz F, Harter P, Traut A, et al. Cerebral metastases (CM) in breast cancer (BC) with focus on triple-negative tumors. J Clin Oncol. 2008;26:abstract 1010.

9. Hammond ME, Hayes DF, Dowsett M, Allred DC, Hagerty KL, Badve S, et al. American Society of Clinical Oncology/College of American Pathologists guideline recommendations for immunohistochemical testing of estrogen and progesterone receptors in breast cancer. Arch Pathol Lab Med. 2010;134(6):907–22.

10. Wolff AC, Hammond ME, Hicks DG, Dowsett M, McShane LM, Allison KH, et al. Recommendations for human epidermal growth factor receptor 2 testing in breast cancer: American Society of Clinical Oncology/College of American Pathologists clinical practice guideline update. Arch Pathol Lab Med. 2014;138(2):241–56.

11. Iwamoto T, Booser D, Valero V, Murray JL, Koenig K, Esteva FJ, et al. Estrogen receptor (ER) mRNA and ER-related gene expression in breast cancers that are 1% to 10% ER-positive by immunohistochemistry. J Clin Oncol. 2012;30(7):729–34.

12. Lehmann BD, Bauer JA, Chen X, Sanders ME, Chakravarthy AB, Shyr Y, et al. Identification of human triple-negative breast cancer subtypes and preclinical models for selection of targeted therapies. J Clin Invest. 2011;121(7):2750–67.

13. Cheang MC, Martin M, Nielsen TO, Prat A, Voduc D, Rodriguez-Lescure A, et al. Defining breast cancer intrinsic subtypes by quantitative receptor expression. Oncologist. 2015;20(5):474–82.

14. Cheang MC, Voduc D, Bajdik C, et al. Basal-like breast cancer defined by five biomarkers has superior prognostic value than triple-negative phenotype. Clin Cancer Res. 2008;14:1368–76.

15. Nielsen TO, Hsu FD, Jensen K, et al. Immunohistochemical and clinical characterization of the basal-like subtype of invasive breast carcinoma. Clin Cancer Res. 2004;10:5367–74.

16. Livasy CA, Karaca G, Nanda R, et al. Phenotypic evaluation of the basal-like subtype of invasive breast carcinoma. Mod Pathol. 2006;19:264–71.

17. Rakha EA, Ellis IO. Triple-negative/basal-like breast cancer: review. Pathology. 2009;41(1):40–7.

18. Subhawong AP, Subhawong T, Nassar H, Kouprina N, Begum S, Vang R, et al. Most basal-like breast carcinomas demonstrate the same Rb−/p16+ immunophenotype as the HPV-related poorly differentiated squamous cell carcinomas which they resemble morphologically. Am J Surg Pathol. 2009;33(2):163–75.

19. Foulkes WD, Smith IE, Reis-Filho JS. Triple-negative breast cancer. N Engl J Med. 2010;363(20):1938–48.

20. Prat A, Parker JS, Karginova O, Fan C, Livasy C, Herschkowitz JI, et al. Phenotypic and molecular characterization of the claudin-low intrinsic subtype of breast cancer. Breast Cancer Res. 2010;12(5):R68.

21. Shah SP, Roth A, Goya R, Oloumi A, Ha G, Zhao Y, et al. The clonal and mutational evolution spectrum of primary triple-negative breast cancers. Nature. 2012;486:395–9.

22. Cancer Genome Atlas Network. Comprehensive molecular portraits of human breast tumours. Nature. 2012;490:61–70.

23. Turner N, Lambros MB, Horlings HM, Pearson A, Sharpe R, Natrajan R, et al. Integrative molecular profiling of triple negative breast cancers identifies amplicon drivers and potential therapeutic targets. Oncogene. 2010;29:2013–23.

24. Stemke-Hale K, Gonzalez-Angulo AM, Lluch A, Neve RM, Kuo WL, Davies M, et al. An integrative genomic and proteomic analysis of PIK3CA, PTEN, and AKT mutations in breast cancer. Cancer Res. 2008;68:6084–91.

25. Putti TC, Abd El-Rahim DM, Rakha EA, et al. Estrogen receptor-negative breast carcinomas: a review of morphology and immunophenotypical analysis. Mod Pathol. 2005;18:26–35.

26. Gaffey MJ, Mills SE, Frierson HF, et al. Medullary carcinoma of the breast: interobserver variability in histopathologic diagnosis. Mod Pathol. 1995;8:31–8.
27. Tsuda H, Takarabe T, Hasegawa F, et al. Large, central acellular zones indicating myoepithelial tumor differentiation in high-grade invasive ductal carcinomas as markers of predisposition to lung and brain metastases. Am J Surg Pathol. 2000;24:197–202.
28. Tsuda H, Takarabe T, Hasegawa T, et al. Myoepithelial differentiation in high-grade ductal carcinomas with large central acellular zones. Hum Pathol. 1999;30:1134–9.
29. Foulkes WE, Brunet JS, Stefaansson IM, et al. The prognostic implication of the basal-like (cyclin E high/p27 low/p53+/glomeruloid-microvascular proliferation+) phenotype of BRCA1-related breast cancer. Cancer Res. 2004;64:356–62.
30. Vazri SA, Krumroy LM, Elson P, et al. Breast tumor immunophenotype of BRCA1-mutation carriers is influenced by age at diagnosis. Clin Cancer Res. 2001;7:1937–45.
31. Foulkes WD, Stefansson IM, Chappuis PO, et al. Germline BRCA1 mutations and a basal epithelial phenotype in breast cancer. J Natl Cancer Inst. 2003;95:1482–5.
32. Lakhani M, Loman N, Borg A, et al. Prediction of BRCA1 status in patients with breast cancer using estrogen receptor and basal phenotype. Clin Cancer Res. 2005;11:5175–80.
33. Farshid G, Balleine RL, Cumming M, et al. Morphology of breast cancer as a means of triage of patients for BRCA1 genetic testing. Am J Surg Pathol. 2006;30:1357–66.
34. Jung SY, Kim HY, Nam BH, Min SY, Lee SJ, Park C, et al. Worse prognosis of metaplastic breast cancer patients than other patients with triple-negative breast cancer. Breast Cancer Res Treat. 2010;120(3):627–37.
35. Chen IC, Lin CH, Huang CS, Lien HC, Hsu C, Kuo WH, et al. Lack of efficacy to systemic chemotherapy for treatment of metaplastic carcinoma of the breast in the modern era. Breast Cancer Res Treat. 2011;130(1):345–51.
36. Ng CKY, Piscuoglio S, Geyer FC, Burke KA, Pareja F, Eberle CA, et al. The landscape of somatic genetic alterations in metaplastic breast carcinomas. Clin Cancer Res. 2017;23:3859.
37. Rosen PP, Ernsberger D. Low-grade adenosquamous carcinoma. A variant of metaplastic mammary carcinoma. Am J Surg Pathol. 1987;11(5):351–8.
38. Sneige N, Yaziji H, Mandavilli SR, Perez ER, Ordonez NG, Gown AM, et al. Low-grade (fibromatosis-like) spindle cell carcinoma of the breast. Am J Surg Pathol. 2001;25(8):1009–16.
39. Gobbi H, Simpson JF, Borowsky A, Jensen RA, Page DL. Metaplastic breast tumors with a dominant fibromatosis-like phenotype have a high risk of local recurrence. Cancer. 1999;85(10):2170–82.
40. Mossler JA, Barton TK, Brinkhous AD, McCarty KS, Moylan JA, McCarty KS Jr. Apocrine differentiation in human mammary carcinoma. Cancer. 1980;46(11):2463–71.
41. Vranic S, Tawfik O, Palazzo J, Bilalovic N, Eyzaguirre E, Lee LM, et al. EGFR and HER-2/neu expression in invasive apocrine carcinoma of the breast. Mod Pathol. 2010;23(5):644–53.
42. Vranic S, Schmitt F, Sapino A, Costa JL, Reddy S, Castro M, et al. Apocrine carcinoma of the breast: a comprehensive review. Histol Histopathol. 2013;28(11):1393–409.
43. Vranic S, Marchio C, Castellano I, Botta C, Scalzo MS, Bender RP, et al. Immunohistochemical and molecular profiling of histologically defined apocrine carcinomas of the breast. Hum Pathol. 2015;46(9):1350–9.
44. Dreyer G, Vandorpe T, Smeets A, Forceville K, Brouwers B, Neven P, et al. Triple negative breast cancer: clinical characteristics in the different histological subtypes. Breast. 2013;22(5):761–6.
45. Nagao T, Kinoshita T, Hojo T, Tsuda H, Tamura K, Fujiwara Y. The differences in the histological types of breast cancer and the response to neoadjuvant chemotherapy: the relationship between the outcome and the clinicopathological characteristics. Breast. 2012;21(3):289–95.
46. Ghabach B, Anderson WF, Curtis RE, et al. Adenoid cystic carcinoma of the breast in the United States (1977 to 2006): a population-based cohort study. Breast Cancer Res. 2010;12:R54.
47. Coates JM, Martinez SR, Bold RJ, Chen SL. Adjuvant radiation therapy is associated with improved survival for adenoid cystic carcinoma of the breast. J Surg Oncol. 2010;102:342–7.

48. Thompson K, Grabowski J, Saltzstein SL, et al. Adenoid cystic breast carcinoma: is axillary staging necessary in all cases? Results from the California Cancer Registry. Breast J. 2011;17:485–9.
49. Ro JY, Silva EG, Gallager HS. Adenoid cystic carcinoma of the breast. Hum Pathol. 1987;18:1276–81.
50. Kleer CG, Oberman HA. Adenoid cystic carcinoma of the breast: value of histologic grading and proliferative activity. Am J Surg Pathol. 1998;22:569–75.
51. Shin SJ, Rosen PP. Solid variant of mammary adenoid cystic carcinoma with basaloid features: a study of nine cases. Am J Surg Pathol. 2002;26:413–20.
52. Brill LB 2nd, Kanner WA, Fehr A, et al. Analysis of MYB expression and MYB-NFIB gene fusions in adenoid cystic carcinoma and other salivary neoplasms. Mod Pathol. 2011;24:1169–76.
53. West RB, Kong C, Clarke N, et al. MYB expression and translocation in adenoid cystic carcinomas and other salivary gland tumors with clinicopathologic correlation. Am J Surg Pathol. 2011;35:92–9.
54. Persson M, Andren Y, Moskaluk CA, et al. Clinically significant copy number alterations and complex rearrangements of MYB and NFIB in head and neck adenoid cystic carcinoma. Genes Chromosomes Cancer. 2012;51:805–17.
55. Wetterskog D, Lopez-Garcia MA, Lambros MB, et al. Adenoid cystic carcinomas constitute a genomically distinct subgroup of triple-negative and basal-like breast cancers. J Pathol. 2012;226:84–96.
56. Martelotto LG, De Filippo MR, Ng CK, et al. Genomic landscape of adenoid cystic carcinoma of the breast. J Pathol. 2015;237:179–89.
57. Lawrence MS, Stojanov P, Polak P, et al. Mutational heterogeneity in cancer and the search for new cancer-associated genes. Nature. 2013;499:214–8.
58. Natrajan R, Lambros MB, Rodriguez-Pinilla SM, et al. Tiling path genomic profiling of grade 3 invasive ductal breast cancers. Clin Cancer Res. 2009;15:2711–22.
59. Natrajan R, Lambros MB, Geyer FC, et al. Loss of 16q in high grade breast cancer is associated with estrogen receptor status: evidence for progression in tumors with a luminal phenotype? Genes Chromosomes Cancer. 2009;48:351–65.
60. Arpino G, Clark GM, Mohsin S, et al. Adenoid cystic carcinoma of the breast: molecular markers, treatment, and clinical outcome. Cancer. 2002;94:2119–27.
61. McDivitt RW, Stewart FW. Breast carcinoma in children. JAMA. 1966;195(5):388–90.
62. Gupta K, Lallu SD, Fauck R, Simpson JS, Wakefield SJ. Needle aspiration cytology, immunocytochemistry, and electron microscopy in a rare case of secretory carcinoma of the breast in an elderly woman. Diagn Cytopathol. 1992;8(4):388–91.
63. Noh WC, Paik NS, Cho KJ, Chung JH, Kim MS, Moon NM. Breast mass in a 3-year-old girl: differentiation of secretory carcinoma versus abnormal thelarche by fine needle aspiration biopsy. Surgery. 2005;137(1):109–10.
64. Tognon C, Knezevich SR, Huntsman D, Roskelley CD, Melnyk N, Mathers JA, et al. Expression of the ETV6-NTRK3 gene fusion as a primary event in human secretory breast carcinoma. Cancer Cell. 2002;2(5):367–76.
65. Strauss BL, Bratthauer GL, Tavassoli FA. STAT 5a expression in the breast is maintained in secretory carcinoma, in contrast to other histologic types. Hum Pathol. 2006;37(5):586–92.
66. Oberman HA. Secretory carcinoma of the breast in adults. Am J Surg Pathol. 1980;4(5):465–70.
67. Oberman HA, Stephens PJ. Carcinoma of the breast in childhood. Cancer. 1972;30(2):470–4.
68. Din NU, Idrees R, Fatima S, Kayani N. Secretory carcinoma of breast: clinicopathologic study of 8 cases. Ann Diagn Pathol. 2013;17(1):54–7.
69. Krausz T, Jenkins D, Grontoft O, Pollock DJ, Azzopardi JG. Secretory carcinoma of the breast in adults: emphasis on late recurrence and metastasis. Histopathology. 1989;14(1):25–36.
70. Byrne MP, Fahey MM, Gooselaw JG. Breast cancer with axillary metastasis in an eight and one-half-year-old girl. Cancer. 1973;31(3):726–8.
71. Tavassoli FA, Norris HJ. Secretory carcinoma of the breast. Cancer. 1980;45(9):2404–13.

72. Herz H, Cooke B, Goldstein D. Metastatic secretory breast cancer. Non-responsiveness to chemotherapy: case report and review of the literature. Ann Oncol. 2000;11(10):1343–7.
73. Aaltomaa S, Lipponen P, Eskelinen M, Kosma VM, Marin S, Alhava E, et al. Lymphocyte infiltrates as a prognostic variable in female breast cancer. Eur J Cancer. 1992;28A(4–5):859–64.
74. Adams S, Gray RJ, Demaria S, Goldstein L, Perez EA, Shulman LN, et al. Prognostic value of tumor-infiltrating lymphocytes in triple-negative breast cancers from two phase III randomized adjuvant breast cancer trials: ECOG 2197 and ECOG 1199. J Clin Oncol. 2014;32(27):2959–66.
75. Salgado R, Denkert C, Demaria S, Sirtaine N, Klauschen F, Pruneri G, et al. The evaluation of tumor-infiltrating lymphocytes (TILs) in breast cancer: recommendations by an International TILs Working Group 2014. Ann Oncol. 2015;26(2):259–71.
76. van de Rijn M, Perou CM, Tibshirani R, et al. Expression of cytokeratins 17 and 5 identifies a group of carcinomas associated with poor clinical outcome. Am J Pathol. 2002;161:1991–6.
77. Abd El-Rehim DM, Pinder SE, Paish CE, et al. Expression of basal and luminal cytokeratins in human breast carcinoma. J Pathol. 2004;203:661–71.
78. Rodriguez-Pinilla SM, Sarrio D, Honrado E, et al. Vimentin and laminin expression is associated with basal-like phenotype in both sporadic and BRCA1-associated breast carcinomas. J Clin Pathol. 2007;60(9):1006–12.
79. Tsuda H, Morita D, Kimura M, et al. Correlation of KIT and EGFR overexpression with invasive ductal carcinoma of the solid-tubular subtype, nuclear grade 3, and mesenchymal or myoepithelial differentiation. Cancer Sci. 2005;96:48–53. J Clin Pathol 2007;60:1017–23
80. Matos I, Dufloth R, Alvarenga M, et al. p63, cytokeratin 5, and P-cadherin: three molecular markers used to distinguish basal phenotype in breast carcinomas. Virchows Arch. 2005;447:688–94.
81. Koker MM, Kleer CG. p63 expression in breast cancer: a highly sensitive and specific marker of metaplastic carcinoma. Am J Surg Pathol. 2004;28:1506–12.
82. Li H, Cherukuri P, Li N, et al. Nestin is expressed in basal/myoepithelial layer of the mammary gland and is a selective marker of basal epithelial breast tumors. Cancer Res. 2007;67:501–10.
83. Reis-Filho JS, Milanezi F, Silva P, et al. Maspin expression in myoepithelial tumors of the breast. Pathol Res Pract. 2001;197:817–21.
84. Moyano JV, Evans JR, Chen F, et al. AlphaB-crystallin is a novel oncoprotein that predicts poor clinical outcome in breast cancer. J Clin Invest. 2006;116:261–70.
85. Pinilla SM, Honrado E, Hardisson D, et al. Caveolin-1 expression is associated with a basal-like phenotype in sporadic and hereditary breast cancer. Breast Cancer Res Treat. 2006;99:85–90.
86. Arnes JB, Brunet JS, Stefansson I, et al. Placental cadherin and the basal epithelial phenotype of BRCA1-related breast cancer. Clin Cancer Res. 2005;11:4003–11.
87. Rodriguez-Pinilla SM, Sarrio D, Honrado E, Hardisson D, Calero F, Benitez J, et al. Prognostic significance of basal-like phenotype and fascin expression in node-negative invasive breast carcinomas. Clin Cancer Res. 2006;12(5):1533–9.
88. Yoder BJ, Tso E, Skacel M, Pettay J, Tarr S, Budd T, et al. The expression of fascin, an actin-bundling motility protein, correlates with hormone receptor-negative breast cancer and a more aggressive clinical course. Clin Cancer Res. 2005;11(1):186–92.
89. Savage K, Leung S, Todd SK, Brown LA, Jones RL, Robertson D, et al. Distribution and significance of caveolin 2 expression in normal breast and invasive breast cancer: an immunofluorescence and immunohistochemical analysis. Breast Cancer Res Treat. 2008;110(2):245–56.
90. Melchor L, Honrado E, Garcia MJ, Alvarez S, Palacios J, Osorio A, et al. Distinct genomic aberration patterns are found in familial breast cancer associated with different immunohistochemical subtypes. Oncogene. 2008;27(22):3165–75.
91. Resetkova E, Reis-Filho JS, Jain RK, Mehta R, Thorat MA, Nakshatri H, et al. Prognostic impact of ALDH1 in breast cancer: a story of stem cells and tumor microenvironment. Breast Cancer Res Treat. 2010;123(1):97–108.
92. Klingbeil P, Natrajan R, Everitt G, Vatcheva R, Marchio C, Palacios J, et al. CD44 is overexpressed in basal-like breast cancers but is not a driver of 11p13 amplification. Breast Cancer Res Treat. 2010;120(1):95–109.

93. Dill EA, Gru AA, Atkins KA, Friedman LA, Moore ME, Bullock TN, et al. PD-L1 expression and intratumoral heterogeneity across breast cancer subtypes and stages: an assessment of 245 primary and 40 metastatic tumors. Am J Surg Pathol. 2017;41(3):334–42.
94. Zhang M, Sun H, Zhao S, Wang Y, Pu H, Wang Y, et al. Expression of PD-L1 and prognosis in breast cancer: a meta-analysis. Oncotarget. 2017;8(19):31347–54.
95. McNamara KM, Yoda T, Takagi K, Miki Y, Suzuki T, Sasano H. Androgen receptor in triple negative breast cancer. J Steroid Biochem Mol Biol. 2013;133:66–76.
96. Pristauz G, Petru E, Stacher E, Geigl JB, Schwarzbraun T, Tsybrovskyy O, et al. Androgen receptor expression in breast cancer patients tested for BRCA1 and BRCA2 mutations. Histopathology. 2010;57(6):877–84.
97. Moinfar F, Okcu M, Tsybrovskyy O, Regitnig P, Lax SF, Weybora W, et al. Androgen receptors frequently are expressed in breast carcinomas: potential relevance to new therapeutic strategies. Cancer. 2003;98(4):703–11.

Triple-Negative Breast Cancer: Clinical Features

2

Tira Tan and Rebecca Dent

Clinical Pearls
- Triple-negative breast cancers occur more commonly in younger patients and vary with race, ethnicity, and socioeconomic status.
- Patients with triple-negative breast cancer have an aggressive natural history, with the risk of distant recurrence highest during the first 3–5 years after diagnosis.
- Visceral metastases are more common in triple-negative breast cancer compared to ER-positive breast cancer, and the most frequent sites of distant disease include the lungs and central nervous system.
- The triple-negative breast cancer subtype responds well to cytotoxic chemotherapy with increased rates of pathologic complete response after neoadjuvant chemotherapy, but poorer prognosis compared with non-triple-negative breast cancer, which is a phenomenon referred to as the triple-negative paradox.

2.1   Definition of Triple-Negative Breast Cancer

TNBCs are defined by what they are not, that is, tumors that do not express any of the three prognostic and predictive biomarkers used in routine clinical management: estrogen receptor (ER), progesterone receptor (PR), and human epidermal growth factor receptor type 2 (HER2). Standardization in the assessment of these biomarkers has gone through changes through the years [1]. Current testing guidelines define the lack of ER and PR receptors as $\leq 1\%$ tumor staining on immunohistochemistry (IHC) [2]. The joint publication of guidelines for HER2 testing by the

T. Tan, BSc, MBBS, MRCP • R. Dent, MD, FRCP (✉)
Division of Medical Oncology, National Cancer Centre Singapore, Singapore, Singapore
e-mail: tira.tan.j.y@singhealth.com.sg; rebecca.dent@singhealth.com.sg

© Springer International Publishing AG 2018
A.R. Tan (ed.), *Triple-Negative Breast Cancer*,
https://doi.org/10.1007/978-3-319-69980-6_2

American Society of Clinical Oncology (ASCO) and College of American Pathologists (CAP) was updated in 2013 and provides recommendations for optimal HER2 testing [3].

TNBC has been further divided into subgroups on the basis of histopathological features and/or gene expression profiling highlighting the heterogeneity and complexity of these tumors [4–7]. From a histologic perspective, TNBC also consists of other subtypes such as secretory or adenoid cystic tumors which are relatively less aggressive and metaplastic breast cancers which are high-grade and aggressive tumors. Four distinct intrinsic subtypes (luminal A, luminal B, HER2 enriched, and basal-like) of prognostic and predictive significance, identified using DNA microarray analysis, were first described by Perou and colleagues in 2000 [8]. Of the four, the basal-like tumors typically are of the triple-negative phenotype, and a vast majority (~80%) of TNBCs are of the basal-like subtype [6, 9]. Another classification of TNBC subtypes through gene expression profiling identifies six distinct molecular subtypes (basal-like 1, basal-like 2, immunomodulatory, mesenchymal, mesenchymal stemlike, and luminal androgen receptor) [5]. This was refined into four tumor-specific subtypes (basal-like 1, basal-like 2, mesenchymal, and luminal androgen receptor) following histopathology and laser-capture microdissection which identified infiltrating lymphocytes and tumor-associated stromal cells contributing to the immunomodulatory and mesenchymal stemlike subtypes, respectively [6]. Clinical trials evaluating the various subgroups and the benefits of different treatment strategies are awaited.

2.2   Epidemiology and Risk Factors

Breast cancer is the most frequent cancer in women and the fifth leading cause of cancer death worldwide [10, 11]. Breast cancer remains common regardless of region; however, incidence rates vary globally. For example, incidence rates range from 27 per 100,000 in Middle Africa to 92 per 100,000 in Northern America [11]. About 15–20% of all invasive breast cancers are of the TNBC subtype which corresponds to approximately 170,000 cases of TNBC globally [10, 12–14].

2.2.1   Age, Ethnicity, and Race

TNBC is more common in younger patients [13, 14] and varies according to race and ethnicity. Studies have consistently reported overrepresentation of TNBC among African American women [9, 14, 15]. The Carolina Breast Cancer Study was a population-based, case-controlled study of environmental and molecular determinants of breast cancer risk [9]. Patients with basal-like tumors as defined by IHC markers (ER−, HER2−, cytokeratin 5/6+, and/or HER1+) were more likely to be African American and premenopausal [9]. The prevalence of basal-like breast cancers in African Americans was 26% as compared to 16% in non-African

American cases in the study [9]. The high prevalence was seen mostly in premeno-pausal African American women in whom the prevalence was 39% [9]. Similarly, a population-based study using the California Cancer Registry data identified 12.5% of the eligible breast cancer cases as TNBC. These women were more likely to be young, under the age of 40 [odds ratio (OR) 1.53; 95% confidence interval (CI) 1.37–1.70] and non-Hispanic blacks (OR 1.77; 95% CI 1.59–1.97) [14]. A report of the US Surveillance, Epidemiology, and End Results (SEER) program, a large-scale population-based study of incidence rates for major breast cancer subtypes, further lends support to these statistics [16]. Among the 57,483 cases diagnosed in 2010, 6193 (12.2%) are of the TNBC subtype. Non-Hispanic black women were more likely to be diagnosed with TNBC than other racial groups (OR = 2.0, 95% CI 1.8–2.2) [16]. In this study, Hispanics were 30% (OR = 1.3, 95% CI 1.2–1.6) more likely to be diagnosed with TNBC as compared to non-Hispanic whites [16]. Age of onset of TNBC is earlier as compared to ER+/HER2− breast cancers. Those diagnosed with TNBC were 10–30% less likely to be aged 65 years and older [16].

Consistent with data from American studies, a high prevalence of TNBC has been reported in Mexico where patients with breast cancer are reported to be younger at time of disease onset [17, 18]. In a retrospective review of 2074 Hispanic breast cancer patients seen between 1998 and 2008 at the National Cancer Institute in Mexico City, the prevalence of TNBC was 23.1% and in univariate analysis, associated with younger age (49.2 vs. 52.2 years; $P < 0.001$) and premenopausal status (OR, 0.72; 95% CI 0.58–0.88; $P = 0.002$), and the latter remained significantly associated with TNBC diagnosis in multivariate analysis [18]. Elsewhere in the world and similar associations for women of African ancestry have also been shown. A study of 507 breast cancer patients in Nigeria and Senegal reports a low mean age of 44.8 years at diagnosis and a majority of tumors being TNBC subtype (27%) [19, 20].

2.2.2   Socioeconomic Status

Typically, the percentage of all breast cancers increases as socioeconomic status increases [14]. However, low socioeconomic status has been associated with breast tumors which are of high-grade, high clinical stage, and ER-negative status. Studies have reported higher odds of TNBC with lower socioeconomic status with some suggestions that the higher odds for TNBC in minority race or ethnic groups is explained by difference in socioeconomic status. Women in areas of low socioeconomic status from the California Cancer Registry were more likely than women living in areas of high socioeconomic status to be diagnosed with TNBC [14].

In a study using data from the National Cancer Data Base (NCDB), a national hospital-based cancer registry involving 260,577 breast cancer cases, the odds of TNBC subtype in minority populations stratified by socioeconomic status was estimated and reported [21]. Consistent with previous results, non-Hispanic blacks had a 1.84 times greater odds (OR = 1.84; 95% CI 1.77–1.92) of having TNBC subtype vs. hormone receptor-positive, HER2-negative subtype compared with non-Hispanic whites [21]. TNBC was also higher in uninsured and Medicaid-insured patients as compared to patients with other insurance types [21]. Patients with low socioeconomic status had a higher proportion of TNBC subtype than other patients and a 1.14 times higher odd of being diagnosed with TNBC subtype (OR = 1.14; 95% CI 1.08–1.19) [21]. In this study, the effect of race or ethnicity of having TNBC is evident even after controlling for difference in socioeconomic status suggesting a role for other factors in the odds differences.

2.2.3   BRCA Mutations

Approximately 5–10% of newly diagnosed breast cancers are attributed to hereditary causes. *BRCA1* and *BRCA2* gene mutations are associated with a 40–60% lifetime risk of female breast cancers [22, 23]. In the general population, deleterious *BRCA1* or *2* mutation rates are approximately 1 in 400 to 1 in 800 people [24]. The prevalence of *BRCA* mutations differs by population groups and ethnicity. For example, approximately 10% of Ashkenazi Jewish women with breast cancer carry a founder mutation in *BRCA1* or *BRCA2* [25, 26]. In a large cross-sectional analysis of 46,276 individuals tested for mutations in *BRCA1* and *BRCA2* genes, women of African ancestry had the highest prevalence of deleterious mutations (15.6% vs. 12.1% for Western European, OR 1.3 (1.1–1.5)) [24]. This group is followed closely by women of Latin American ethnicity with a prevalence of 14.8% vs. 12.1% for Western European (OR 1.2, 95% CI 1.1–1.4). In both groups, the number of *BRCA1* mutations was twice as many as *BRCA2* mutations [24].

It is estimated that 25% of TNBCs carry a *BRCA1* mutation, and more than 75% of tumors in women who carry the *BRCA* gene are of the triple-negative and/or basal-like phenotype [12]. In a retrospective review of 469 subjects with TNBC referred to the hereditary cancer risk clinics at Duke and University of California, San Francisco, 31% tested positive for a mutation in *BRCA1*, *BRCA2*, or both genes [27]. In a study examining *BRCA* mutations in a cohort of young breast and ovarian cancer patients unselected for family history in Mexico, a high prevalence of *BRCA* mutations (9 out of 33 TNBC, 27%) was reported in women with TNBC. All nine harbored a mutation in the *BRCA1* gene [17].

2.2.4   Other Risk Factors: Obesity, Parity, and Breastfeeding

Risk factors of TNBC differ slightly from that of other breast cancer subtypes. In general, a reduction in lifetime exposure to estrogen, long duration of breastfeeding, high parity, and young age at first pregnancy can protect from hormone receptor-positive breast cancers. The risk of TNBC differs slightly and is positively associated with higher parity in addition to being negatively associated with duration of breastfeeding [9, 18, 28, 29]. Women with TNBC had younger ages at menarche and at first full-term pregnancy [29]. Kwan et al. report on data from two large prospective breast cancer survivorship studies. Premenopausal TNBC cases were more likely to be overweight [30].

2.3   Clinical Presentation

Primary TNBC tumors are larger, of higher grade, and grow rapidly [9, 13, 14, 16, 31]. TNBC cancers are more often interval cancers occurring between mammographic screening and are clinically detectable at time of diagnosis [13]. The presence of lymph node metastasis at time of diagnosis of TNBC is conflicting. Dent et al. suggest a higher prevalence of lymph node metastasis in TNBC which does not correlate with tumor size; 55% of women with tumors 1 cm and less in their study had at least one positive lymph node [13]. On the other hand, the Carolina Breast Cancer Study reports no association with positive axillary lymph nodes and basal-like subtype [9]. Upon disease recurrence, a higher proportion of patients with TNBC will experience distant recurrence as compared to local recurrence, and few will experience local recurrence before a distant one [13]. Metastatic TNBCs are more likely to involve the viscera such as the lungs and brains and less likely to involve the bones in contrast to their ER-positive counterpart. The majority of patients will present with multiple sites of disease [12, 32].

2.4   Young vs. Older Triple-Negative Breast Cancer

Approximately 21% of breast cancers are diagnosed at age 70 years and older [11]. Typically, an older age of breast cancer diagnosis is associated with ER-positive breast cancers [14, 16]. However, around 15% of breast cancers in older patients are triple-negative [33]. In a SEER database study investigating the survival pattern of elderly TNBC, older TNBC women had tumors with biologically favorable phenotype. Older TNBC patients tended to have a lower likelihood of lymph node metastases (N0, 69.5% vs. 63.8%; $P < 0.001$), lower TNM stage, and lower tumor grade as compared to younger TNBC patients [34]. Consequently, studies have suggested that older patients with TNBC have similar outcomes when compared with their younger counterparts. In a single institution report of 1759 women aged 70 and above with early operable primary breast cancers, 22% of breast cancers in older women ($\geq$70 years old) were of the TNBC subtypes [35]. There was a clear difference in the management pattern where 47% of patients younger than 70 years old received adjuvant chemotherapy following surgery and no older patient received adjuvant chemotherapy [35]. Despite this, there was a non-statistically significant trend toward better survival in older women [35]. The 5-year breast cancer-specific survival in <70 years was 73% compared to 79% in 70 years and older patients [35]. There was no difference in the 5-year local-regional (local recurrence 10% vs. 14%; regional recurrence 9% vs. 14%) and rates of distant metastases (30% vs. 27%) in the younger and older groups, respectively [35].

2.5   Natural History and Prognosis

TNBCs are aggressive tumors which carry a poorer prognosis as compared to their luminal counterpart [13–15]. For example, in the population-based study from the California Cancer Registry, the relative survival of women with TNBC was poorer as compared to non-TNBC; 77% of women with TNBC were still alive 5 years after diagnosis as compared to 93% for other breast cancers [14]. When compared with women with other breast cancers, women with TNBC had consistently poorer survival for each stage [14]. The median time to death was shorter for patients with TNBC compared to patients with other subtypes [13]. In addition to being more likely to experience distant recurrences, patients with TNBC are also likely to experience recurrences earlier [13]. The mean time to distant recurrence in a cohort of TNBC patients diagnosed at a single institution in Toronto was 2.6 vs. 5 years ($P < 0.0001$) for other tumor types, respectively. The risk of relapse and death for TNBC is highest during the first 3–5 years from diagnosis [9, 13]. After adjusting for known prognostic variables such as age, grade, tumor size, chemotherapy, and nodal status, the risk of death from breast cancer remained higher for TNBC up to 5 years from diagnosis with a hazard ratio of 1.8 (95% confidence interval (CI) 1.2–2.6; $P = 0.0005$) [13]. This increase was not observed for the period beyond 5 years after diagnosis. All TNBC deaths occur earlier and within 10 years of diagnosis. In contrast, death from breast cancer in patients with other cancer subtypes continues to accrue for up to 18 years after diagnosis [13]. This pattern of recurrence is illustrated by the BEATRICE trial [36]. To date, this trial has enrolled the largest cohort of TNBC patients and evaluates the use of 1 year of bevacizumab in addition to standard chemotherapy in TNBC. A total of 2591 patients were enrolled from 37 countries, and about two thirds of the patients had node-negative disease. The 3-year invasive disease-free survival (DFS) was 83% with distant recurrence in 11% of patient. The most frequent sites of distant recurrences were the lungs (~30%), liver (15–20%), and bone (~20%). Distant CNS recurrence accounted for approximately 7–12% of distant recurrences. Following metastasis, patients with TNBC have a shorter survival as compared to non-TNBC, and the median survival time from diagnosis of distant metastatic disease was 9 vs. 22 months in the cohort of 1601 patients with breast cancer as reported by Dent et al. [13]. Contemporary TNBC studies have reported a median survival time from diagnosis of metastatic disease of around 1 year which unfortunately remains relatively unchanged for the past decade [32].

2.6   Treatment and the Triple-Negative Paradox

There are currently no targeted therapies approved for use in TNBC. Chemotherapy is the mainstay of treatment to which some TNBCs are exquisitely sensitive. Yet, despite sensitivity to chemotherapy, TNBC is still associated with a poor prognosis otherwise described as the triple-negative paradox. In a retrospective cohort study examining the relationship between response to neoadjuvant chemotherapy, long-term end points, and breast cancer subtypes, Carey and colleagues report a high clinical response rate of 85% for TNBC to anthracycline-based chemotherapy as compared to the luminal subtypes with a response rate of 39–58% [37]. Pathological complete response to chemotherapy was significantly higher in TNBC (27%) as compared to the luminal subtypes (7%) [37]. Despite this, there was a significant difference in 4-year distant disease-free survival of 71% (95% CI 51–84%) vs. 82%

(95% CI 64–91%) [37]. The poorer outcome is contributed predominantly by those with residual disease following neoadjuvant chemotherapy who had a worse survival due to high early relapse rates resulting in death [37]. The particularly poor outcomes of TNBC patients with residual cancer post-neoadjuvant chemotherapy lend support to efforts focusing on this challenging group of patients. Notably, CREATE-X, a study of adjuvant capecitabine in HER2-negative breast cancers with residual disease post-neoadjuvant therapy, demonstrated an improvement in 5-year DFS 69.8% vs. 56.1% (HR 0.58; 95% CI 0.39–0.87) and overall survival (OS) 78.8% vs. 70.3% (HR 0.52; 95% CI 0.30–0.90) in the cohort of TNBC patients [38].

Several clinical trials evaluating novel treatment strategies in metastatic TNBC are ongoing. Clinical experience suggests that many women with metastatic TNBC relapse and progress quickly on chemotherapy. In a retrospective chart review of patients with metastatic TNBC who received first-line chemotherapy, duration of first-, second-, and third-line chemotherapy was used as a surrogate for duration of treatment response [32]. The median duration of first-line chemotherapy for all patients was 11.9 weeks (range 0–73.1 weeks), and 78% of patients went on to receive second-line chemotherapy with a median duration of 9 weeks (range 0–120.9 weeks), and 49% received third-line chemotherapy with a median duration of 3 weeks (0–59 weeks) [32]. Multivariate analysis revealed five predictors of survival which included history of previous adjuvant or neoadjuvant chemotherapy (HR 2.77; 95% CI 1.39–5.52; $P = 0.004$), distant disease-free interval >12 months (HR 0.36, 95% CI 0.26–0.83; $P = 0.01$), age >50 at diagnosis of metastatic disease (HR 0.46, 95% CI 0.27–0.76; $P = 0.003$), type of metastatic disease (visceral vs. non-visceral) (HR 1.94; $P = 0.021$), and increased alkaline phosphatase levels (HR 2.4; $P = 0.002$). It is important to take the aggressive and progressive nature of this disease and the short window for therapeutic intervention into account. This represents a challenge in the clinical management of these patients as physicians treat to palliate and extend life and also in the design of clinical trials that either focus or include this poor-risk group. As an example, in KEYNOTE-086, a phase II study of single-agent pembrolizumab, a fully human IgG4 monoclonal antibody that directly blocks the interaction between the T-cell inhibitory molecule programmed death receptor-1 (PD-1) and its ligands, programmed death-ligand 1 (PD-L1) and programmed death-ligand 2 (PD-L2), for previously treated metastatic TNBC, 386 patients were screened to enroll 170 patients resulting in a high screen fail rate of more than 50% [39]. Secondly, the high response rates and yet poorer outcomes of TNBC calls to question the use of response rate as a surrogate end point. Finally, with technological advances in interrogating the genome, transcriptome, and proteome, we see a shift in the paradigm of cancer care as we move toward precision medicine. Novel trial designs such as umbrella and basket trials can enroll patients with companion molecular marker testing and assess the efficacy of treatment for the identified marker. An important goal in all trials is to identify prognostic and predictive factors to reliably select TNBC patients for different treatment approaches. Important limitations of studying this poor-risk population need to be overcome, and identifying TNBC patients for select trial needs to be performed expeditiously and ideally early during the course of their metastatic disease.

Conclusion

The natural history of TNBC has been described over the past 15 years consequent to the refinement of breast cancer subtypes. Moving forward, integration of molecular data will shed light on the TNBC subtype biology as well as treatment for early and late disease. At the individual patient level of care, what is needed is to integrate the pathological, clinical, and molecular data with encouragement of enrollment onto clinical trials to optimize care. Additionally, increasing attention to germline risk factors for the development of TNBC will enhance early detection and improve survival.

References

1. Allred DC. Issues and updates: evaluating estrogen receptor-alpha, progesterone receptor, and HER2 in breast cancer. Mod Pathol. 2010;23(Suppl 2 (S2)):S52–9.
2. Hammond MEH, Hayes DF, Dowsett M, Allred DC, Hagerty KL, Badve S, et al. American Society of Clinical Oncology/College of American Pathologists guideline recommendations for immunohistochemical testing of estrogen and progesterone receptors in breast cancer. Arch Pathol Lab Med. 2010;134(6):907–22.
3. Wolff AC, Hammond ME, Hicks DG, Dowsett M, McShane LM, Allison KH, et al. Recommendations for human epidermal growth factor receptor 2 testing in breast cancer: American Society of Clinical Oncology/College of American Pathologists clinical practice guideline update. J Clin Oncol. 2013;31 VN-r(31):3997–4013.
4. Penault-Llorca F, Viale G. Pathological and molecular diagnosis of triple-negative breast cancer: a clinical perspective. Ann Oncol. 2012;23(Suppl. 6):vi19–22.
5. Lehmann BD, Bauer JA, Chen X, Sanders ME, Chakravarthy AB, Shyr Y, et al. Identification of human triple-negative breast cancer subtypes and preclinical models for selection of targeted therapies. J Clin Invest. 2011;121(7):2750–67.
6. Lehmann BD, Jovanović B, Chen X, Estrada MV, Johnson KN, Shyr Y, et al. Refinement of triple-negative breast cancer molecular subtypes: implications for neoadjuvant chemotherapy selection. PLoS One. 2016;11(6):1–22.
7. Burstein MD, Tsimelzon A, Poage GM, Covington KR, Contreras A, Fuqua S, et al. Comprehensive genomic analysis identifies novel subtypes and targets of triple-negative breast cancer. Clin Cancer Res. 2014;21(i):1688–99.
8. Perou CM, Sørlie T, Eisen MB, van de Rijn M, Jeffrey SS, Rees CA, et al. Molecular portraits of human breast tumours. Nature. 2000;406(6797):747–52.
9. Carey LA, Perou CM, Livasy CA, Dressler LG, Cowan D, Conway K, et al. Race, breast cancer subtypes, and survival in the Carolina Breast Cancer Study. JAMA. 2006;295(21):2492.
10. Boyle P. Triple-negative breast cancer: epidemiological considerations and recommendations. Ann Oncol. 2012;23(Suppl. 6):8–13.
11. Ferlay J, Soerjomataram I, Ervik M, Dikshit R, Eser S, Mathers C, Rebelo M, Parkin DM, Forman D, Bray F. GLOBOCAN 2012 v1.0, cancer incidence and mortality worldwide: IARC CancerBase No. 11. International Agency for Research on Cancer: Lyon; 2013.
12. Foulkes WD, Smith IE, Reis-Filho JS. Triple-negative breast cancer. N Engl J Med. 2010;363:1938–48.
13. Dent R, Trudeau M, Pritchard KI, Hanna WM, Kahn HK, Sawka CA, et al. Triple-negative breast cancer: clinical features and patterns of recurrence. Clin Cancer Res. 2007;13(15):4429–34.
14. Bauer KR, Brown M, Cress RD, Parise CA, Caggiano V. Descriptive analysis of estrogen receptor (ER)-negative, progesterone receptor (PR)-negative, and HER2-negative invasive breast cancer, the so-called triple-negative phenotype: a population-based study from the California cancer Registry. Cancer. 2007;109(9):1721–8.

15. Harris LN, Broadwater G, Lin NU, Miron A, Schnitt SJ, Cowan D, et al. Molecular subtypes of breast cancer in relation to paclitaxel response and outcomes in women with metastatic disease: results from CALGB 9342. Breast Cancer Res. 2006;8(6):R66.
16. Howlader N, Altekruse SF, Li CI, Chen VW, Clarke CA, Ries LAG, et al. US incidence of breast cancer subtypes defined by joint hormone receptor and HER2 status. J Natl Cancer Inst. 2014;106(5). pii: dju055.
17. Villarreal-Garza C, Alvarez-Gómez RM, Pérez-Plasencia C, Herrera LA, Herzog J, Castillo D, et al. Significant clinical impact of recurrent BRCA1 and BRCA2 mutations in Mexico. Cancer. 2015;121(3):372–8.
18. Lara-Medina F, Pérez-Sánchez V, Saavedra-Pérez D, Blake-Cerda M, Arce C, Motola-Kuba D, et al. Triple-negative breast cancer in Hispanic patients: high prevalence, poor prognosis, and association with menopausal status, body mass index, and parity. Cancer. 2011;117(16):3658–69.
19. Brewster AM, Chavez-MacGregor M, Brown P. Epidemiology, biology, and treatment of triple-negative breast cancer in women of African ancestry. Lancet Oncol. 2014;15(13):e625–34.
20. Huo D, Ikpatt F, Khramtsov A, Dangou JM, Nanda R, Dignam J, et al. Population differences in breast cancer: survey in indigenous african women reveals over-representation of triple-negative breast cancer. J Clin Oncol. 2009;27(27):4515–21.
21. Sineshaw HM, Gaudet M, Ward EM, Flanders WD, Desantis C, Lin CC, et al. Association of race/ethnicity, socioeconomic status, and breast cancer subtypes in the National Cancer Data Base (2010-2011). Breast Cancer Res Treat. 2014;145(3):753–63.
22. Chen S, Parmigiani G. Meta-analysis of BRCA1 and BRCA2 penetrance. J Clin Oncol. 2007;25(11):1329–33.
23. KB K, JL H, DR B. al et. Risks of breast, ovarian, and contralateral breast cancer for brca1 and brca2 mutation carriers. JAMA. 2017;317(23):2402–16.
24. Hall MJ, Reid JE, Burbidge LA, Pruss D, Deffenbaugh AM, Frye C, et al. BRCA1 and BRCA2 mutations in women of different ethnicities undergoing testing for hereditary breast-ovarian cancer. Cancer. 2009;115(10):2222–33.
25. Comen E, Davids M, Kirchhoff T, Hudis C, Offit K, Robson M. Relative contributions of BRCA1 and BRCA2 mutations to "triple-negative" breast cancer in Ashkenazi Women. Breast Cancer Res Treat. 2011;129(1):185–90.
26. Warner E, Foulkes W, Goodwin P, Meschino W, Blondal J, Paterson C, et al. Prevalence and penetrance of BRCA1 and BRCA2 gene mutations in unselected Ashkenazi Jewish women with breast cancer. J Natl Cancer Inst. 1999;91(14):1241–7.
27. Greenup R, Buchanan A, Lorizio W, Rhoads K, Chan S, Leedom T, et al. Prevalence of BRCA mutations among women with Triple-Negative Breast Cancer (TNBC) in a Genetic Counseling Cohort. Ann Surg Oncol. 2013;20(10):3254–8.
28. Millikan RC, Newman B, Tse CK, Moorman PG, Conway K, Smith LV, et al. Epidemiology of basal-like breast cancer. Breast Cancer Res Treat. 2008;109(1):123–39.
29. Shinde SS, Forman MR, Kuerer HM, Yan K, Peintinger F, Hunt KK, et al. Higher parity and shorter breastfeeding duration. Cancer. 2010;116(21):4933–43.
30. Kwan ML, Kushi LH, Weltzien E, Maring B, Kutner SE, Fulton RS, et al. Epidemiology of breast cancer subtypes in two prospective cohort studies of breast cancer survivors. Breast Cancer Res. 2009;11(3):R31.
31. Reis-Filho JS, Tutt ANJ. Triple negative tumours: a critical review. Histopathology. 2008;52(1):108–18.
32. Kassam F, Enright K, Dent R, Dranitsaris G, Myers J, Flynn C, et al. Survival outcomes for patients with metastatic triple-negative breast cancer: implications for clinical practice and trial design. Clin Breast Cancer. 2009;9(1):29–33.
33. Aapro M, Wildiers H. Triple-negative breast cancer in the older population. Ann Oncol. 2012;23(Suppl. 6):vi52–5.
34. Zhu W, Perez EA, Hong R, Li Q, Xu B. Age-related disparity in immediate prognosis of patients with triple-negative breast cancer: a population-based study from SEER cancer registries. PLoS One. 2015;10(5):1–15.

35. Syed BM, Green AR, Nolan CC, Morgan DAL, Ellis IO, Cheung KL. Biological characteristics and clinical outcome of triple negative primary breast cancer in older women – comparison with their younger counterparts. PLoS One. 2014;9(7):e100573.
36. Cameron D, Brown J, Dent R, Jackisch C, Mackey J, Pivot X, et al. Adjuvant bevacizumab-containing therapy in triple-negative breast cancer (BEATRICE): primary results of a randomised, phase 3 trial. Lancet Oncol. 2013;14(10):933–42.
37. Carey LA, Dees EC, Sawyer L, Gatti L, Moore DT, Collichio F, et al. The triple negative paradox: primary tumor chemosensitivity of breast cancer subtypes. Clin Cancer Res. 2007;13(8):2329–34.
38. Masuda N, Lee S-J, Ohtani S, Im Y-H, Lee E-S, Yokota I, et al. Adjuvant capecitabine for breast cancer after preoperative chemotherapy. N Engl J Med. 2017;376(22):2147–59.
39. Adams S, Schmid P, Rugo HS, Winer EP, Loirat D, Awada A, et al. Phase 2 study of pembrolizumab (pembro) monotherapy for previously treated metastatic triple-negative breast cancer (mTNBC): KEYNOTE-086 cohort A. American Society of Clinical Oncology Annual Meeting; 2017.

The Genetics of Triple-Negative Breast Cancer

3

Nanna H. Sulai and Olufunmilayo I. Olopade

Clinical Pearls
- Approximately 11–20% of patients with triple-negative breast cancer unselected for family history harbor a *BRCA1* or *BRCA2* mutation.
- Germline *BRCA1* mutations are more frequently associated with triple-negative breast cancer than *BRCA2* mutations.
- About 70% of *BRCA1*-associated breast cancers are triple-negative.
- Patients diagnosed with triple-negative breast cancer ≤60 years of age should be referred for genetic counseling and testing.
- Poly (ADP-ribose) polymerase inhibitors show antitumor activity in advanced HER2-negative breast cancer with *BRCA* mutations.

3.1 Implicated Genes in Triple-Negative Breast Cancer

BRCA1 and *BRCA2* are the two major cancer susceptibility genes that contribute to inherited breast cancer. In fact, an inherited *BRCA1* mutation is the strongest predictor of triple-negative breast cancer (TNBC). The *BRCA1* gene was identified in 1994 and mapped to chromosome 17 [1], and *BRCA2* was mapped to chromosome 13 [2]. Both genes are involved in repairing double-strand DNA breaks [3]. *BRCA1* and *BRCA2* mutation carriers are associated with a cumulative breast cancer risk to age 80 of 72% and 69%, respectively. The risk of developing contralateral breast

N.H. Sulai, MD (✉)
Department of Solid Tumor Oncology and Investigational Therapeutics,
Levine Cancer Institute, Carolinas HealthCare System, Charlotte, NC, USA
e-mail: nanna.sulai@carolinashealthcare.org

O.I. Olopade, MD, FACP
Department of Internal Medicine, Division of Hematology Oncology, University of Chicago
Medical Center, Chicago, IL, USA
e-mail: folopade@medicine.bsd.uchicago.edu

© Springer International Publishing AG 2018
A.R. Tan (ed.), *Triple-Negative Breast Cancer*,
https://doi.org/10.1007/978-3-319-69980-6_3

cancer 20 years after an initial diagnosis is estimated at 40% for *BRCA1* and 26% for *BRCA2*. The cumulative ovarian cancer risk to age 80 years was estimated at 44% for *BRCA1* and 17% for *BRCA2* carriers [4].

Several studies suggest that 50–70% of *BRCA1*-associated breast cancer is triple-negative [5–7]. In contrast, among *BRCA2* mutation carriers, only 16% of tumors are triple-negative [7]. A meta-analysis of 12 studies with over 2533 breast cancer patients from a high-risk population showed that women with TNBC are greater than five and a half times (RR 5.65; 95% CI, 4.15–7.69) more likely to have a *BRCA1* mutation compared to non-triple-negative patients [8]. Reported frequency of *BRCA1* mutations among triple-negative patients ranges from 8 to 28% [9–11]. In an analysis of 284 women diagnosed with TNBC, 30 deleterious mutations in *BRCA1* were seen in 10% of the patients, thus estimating that BRCA1 mutation accounted for 10.6% of the cases [12]. Among the 30 carriers, 10 women had no family history of breast or ovarian cancer which confirms the importance of testing women with TNBC even in the absence of a family history of cancer. The incidence of underlying germline *BRCA* mutations was studied in an unselected 77 patient population from a single institution where a 19.5% incidence of *BRCA* mutations were seen. *BRCA1* mutations were seen in 12 patients and *BRCA2* mutations in 3 patients [13].

3.2   Characteristics of *BRCA*-Associated Triple-Negative Breast Cancer

The characteristics of TNBC in patients with a *BRCA1* mutation include younger age at diagnosis with a median age of 39 years [12, 13]. For patients with TNBC diagnosed before 40 years, *BRCA1* mutations were found in 36–47% of patients [11, 12]. The *BRCA1* mutation frequency among patients with TNBC seems to decrease with age with estimated frequency of 3.5–7.7% in women >60 years of age [14].

Higher tumor grade and greater tumor stage are also observed in TNBC patients with *BRCA1* mutations [5, 11]. Women with *BRCA1* mutation who developed TNBC also had a higher premenopausal body mass index and earlier age of first birth compared to those who did not develop TNBC. In addition, the development of TNBC was five times higher in *BRCA1* mutation carriers who were Ashkenazi Jewish women, compared to those who were not [5].

3.3   Ethnic Variations of *BRCA* Mutations and Associated Breast Cancer

The proportion of breast cancer cases due to *BRCA1* and *BRCA2* mutations vary depending on the ancestral group. Among TNBC cases, *BRCA1* and *BRCA2* mutation frequencies vary by ethnicity and how the cases were ascertained. In a genetic counseling cohort of TNBC cases, mutation prevalence was quite high depending on the race and ethnicity of the proband with a prevalence of 50% in Ashkenazi Jewish women, 22.2% in Caucasian women, and 20.4% in African American women [15].

The three most common mutations considered the founder mutations among Ashkenazi Jews include *BRCA1*185delAG, *BRCA1*5382insC, and *BRCA2* 6174delT [16]. Approximately 5% of the general population have an underlying *BRCA* mutation. Among Ashkenazi Jewish women with breast cancer, up to 10% have a *BRCA1* mutation and about 2% have a *BRCA2* mutation. The likelihood of an Ashkenazi Jewish woman with breast cancer harboring an underlying *BRCA1/2* mutation is significantly higher when they have TNBC [17].

The lifetime risk of developing breast cancer is highest in black women when compared to Asian, Hispanic, and white counterparts [18]. Black women also tend to have a more aggressive disease associated with earlier ages of onset, higher grade, and advanced stages at presentation [19]. In a pathologic review of over 507 breast cancer patients of African ancestry from Nigeria and Senegal, hormone receptor-negative breast cancer was the most predominant with only 255 identified as ER-positive [19]. While this may explain the poor prognosis associated with breast cancer in developing countries, it does not explain why the difference in molecular subtypes exists. A high frequency of pathogenic mutations may exist in this patient population as an analysis of over 400 Nigerian breast cancer patients identified a 7.1% *BRCA1* and 3.9% *BRCA2* mutation rate [20]. Among a cohort of African American patients with TNBC, 29% had an inherited mutation with the majority involving *BRCA1* or *BRCA2* [21].

3.4 Other Involved Genes Beyond *BRCA1/2*

The advent of rapid, more affordable commercial next generation sequencing studies has changed the landscape of genetic evaluation as multiple genes can now be evaluated all at once. This technology has led to panel testing where more than 100 genes with potential cancer associations can be evaluated, thus providing information on genes beyond *BRCA1/2* [18].

Various population studies have sought to determine the frequency of the most common genetic mutations among patients with TNBC. In an analysis by Couch and colleagues, germline DNA of 1824 patients with TNBC were analyzed [11]. These patients were unselected based on family history of other malignancies including breast and ovarian cancer. Pathogenic mutations were identified in 14.6% of patients of which most of the mutations were in *BRCA1* (57%) and *BRCA2* (18%). About 25% of the mutations were identified in other genes involved in homologous recombination repair such as *PALB2* (7.7%), *BARD1* (3.3%), *RAD51D* (2.5%), *RAD50* (2.2%), and *RAD51C* (2.2%). These moderate penetrance genes are associated with at least a two- to fourfold increase in breast cancer risk [22] and occur commonly in younger onset cases [11]. A similar heterogeneous mutational spectrum was noted in a single institutional study of African American breast cancer patients, in which 22% of 289 patients were found to have germline pathogenic mutations with 57 different mutations identified in 65 patients. Notably, 80% of the mutations were in *BRCA1* or *BRCA2*, and the rest were in *PALB2, CHEK2, BARD1, ATM, PTEN*, or *TP53* [21].

Other known breast cancer predisposing syndromes include Li-Fraumeni syndrome (LFS), Cowden syndrome, Peutz-Jeghers syndrome, and hereditary diffuse gastric cancer syndrome. Among LFS patients which is a syndrome due to a germline mutation in the tumor suppressor protein gene *TP53*, the lifetime breast cancer risk is 49% by age 60 [23]. Early onset breast cancer accounts for 25% of all LFS-associated cancers [24] and is increased by more than a 100-fold among mutation carriers [25]. Among pathologic review of 43 breast cancer tumors from germline *TP53* mutation carriers, the median age of diagnosis was 32 with 75% being invasive ductal adenocarcinoma and ductal carcinoma in situ making up the rest. Only 5% of the cases were triple-negative which confirms that majority of LFS-associated breast cancer is hormone receptor-positive and/or HER2-amplified [23].

3.5   Identification of Pathogenic Mutation Carriers

Advances in genetics have allowed the identification of at-risk women prior to the development of breast cancer. Genetic risk evaluation performed by a qualified cancer genetics risk expert should be offered to individuals who have a high risk of disease for which management recommendations can be implemented to decrease their risk. A detailed assessment will consist of assessing the patient's needs and concerns regarding the anticipated goal of familial risk assessment, obtaining a detailed family history, and reviewing existing medical history and gynecologic risk factors which contribute to the development of breast cancer such as parity, age of menarche, oral contraceptive use, and performing a focused physical exam.

Several consensus guidelines including the National Comprehensive Cancer Network (NCCN) and the American Society of Clinical Oncology (ASCO) have been developed to identify and manage high-risk individuals. Genetic testing should be offered to an individual without a personal history of breast cancer if there is a family history of a known cancer predisposing mutation, multiple relatives with breast cancer with one diagnosed <50 years, or a family history of other malignancies including ovarian cancer, melanoma, diffuse gastric cancer, colon cancer, endometrial cancer, pancreatic cancer, or prostate cancer. The criteria for genetic testing in breast cancer patients include any individual with TNBC at ≤60 years of age, breast cancer in a patient with a family history of a known mutation in a cancer-predisposing gene, early age onset of breast cancer diagnosed at ≤50 years of age, a patient with multiple breast cancer primaries, and breast cancer at any age with a family history of early onset breast cancer, ovarian cancer, or pancreatic cancer [26–28].

3.6   High-Risk Breast Cancer Screening and Prevention

The NCCN and the American Cancer Society recommend the addition of annual bilateral breast MRI in addition to annual breast mammogram for women who have a breast cancer lifetime risk of 20% or greater. One's risk is calculated using several models which incorporate family and personal risk factors [29]. Women with underlying *BRCA1/2* mutations qualify since their lifetime risk exceeds 20% and should begin MRI screening by age 25 and mammograms at age 30 [30, 31]. Mutation carriers of *ATM, CHEK2, NBN,* and *PALB2* also qualify for breast MRI screening since their cumulative lifetime risk is greater than 20% [22]. The extent of the lifetime risk associated with some penetrance genes is unclear, such as *RAD51C* and *BARD1*, and as such MRI is not recommended in these cases [10].

Once a pathogenic *BRCA* mutation is identified, the management involves more intensive screening and/or risk-reducing procedures. Breast cancer risk screening involves clinical breast exams every 6–12 months starting at age 25. In addition, annual mammograms starting at age 30 with annual bilateral breast MRIs starting at age 25–29 years should be performed and are spaced 6 months apart [32]. A prophylactic mastectomy is recommended for *BRCA1/2* mutation carriers which is highly effective for primary prevention of cancer, as it reduces the risk of breast cancer by 90% [33]. It is also acceptable to continue with more intensive breast cancer screening [22]. Annual transvaginal ultrasounds and annual evaluation of the tumor marker CA125 are used to monitor for ovarian cancer. These tests are not highly sensitive or specific [34]. Consequently, a risk-reducing salpingo-oophorectomy (RRSO) between the ages of 35 and 40 is also recommended to be performed while premenopausal. A RRSO can be later between the ages of 40 and 45 for *BRCA2* patients provided patients have undergone bilateral prophylactic mastectomy. RRSO has been demonstrated in several studies to lower the risk of ovarian and fallopian cancer by 80–85% [35, 36]. The management of patients with other less commonly affected genes continues to evolve. The identification of hereditary mutations is important because it empowers affected individuals to undergo risk-reducing strategies and identifies family members of those affected who are yet to develop cancer and can engage in active cancer prevention.

3.7   Treatment of Triple-Negative Breast Cancer with Hereditary Risk

While TNBC responds to currently available chemotherapy regimens, the inability to treat with targeted agents makes it challenging. Most patients diagnosed with advanced TNBC are treated with multiple chemotherapy regimens, become refractory to treatment, and experience higher rates of visceral and central nervous system metastases [37, 38].

Poly (ADP-ribose) polymerase (PARP) inhibitors have shown activity in breast cancer patients with inherited mutations in the *BRCA* pathway. OlympiAD is a randomized phase III study that evaluated the efficacy of olaparib, an oral PARP inhibitor, compared to chemotherapy of physician's choice, which included capecitabine, eribulin, or vinorelbine, in 302 patients with metastatic HER2-negative *BRCA*-associated breast cancer [39]. The median progression-free survival was longer in the olaparib-treated group than in the chemotherapy-treated group (7.0 vs. 4.2 months; HR 0.58, 95% CI 0.43–0.80; $P < 0.001$). In the group as a whole, the response rate was 59.9% with olaparib treatment and 28.8% with chemotherapy. In the triple-negative subgroup, the response rate was better with olaparib compared to chemotherapy (54.7% vs. 21.2%). Future studies are ongoing to assess the long term of outcome from treatment with PARP inhibitors. These drugs have biological and clinical activity as a single agent in the treatment of *BRCA1/2*-associated advanced TNBC.

Conclusion

A subgroup of TNBCs is due to inherited mutations with the majority involving either *BRCA1* or *BRCA2*. Several other genes have been identified with the use of next generation sequencing. Identification of existing germline mutations allows affected individuals to undergo intensive screening and risk-reducing strategies which decrease the likelihood of developing cancer. The treatment of TNBC is evolving with therapies, such as PARP inhibitors, designed to target underlying DNA repair pathways with promising results.

References

1. Miki Y, Swensen J, Shattuck-Eidens D, et al. A strong candidate for the breast and ovarian cancer susceptibility gene BRCA1. Science. 1994;266:66–71.
2. Wooster R, Neuhausen SL, Mangion J, et al. Localization of a breast cancer susceptibility gene, BRCA2, to chromosome 13q12-13. Science. 1994;265:2088–90.
3. Li X, Heyer WD. Homologous recombination in DNA repair and DNA damage tolerance. Cell Res. 2008;18:99–113.
4. Kuchenbaecker KB, Hopper JL, Barnes DR, et al. Risks of breast, ovarian, and contralateral breast cancer for BRCA1 and BRCA2 mutation carriers. JAMA. 2017;317:2402–16.
5. Lee E, McKean-Cowdin R, Ma H, et al. Characteristics of triple-negative breast cancer in patients with a BRCA1 mutation: results from a population-based study of young women. J Clin Oncol. 2011;29:4373–80.
6. Atchley DP, Albarracin CT, Lopez A, et al. Clinical and pathologic characteristics of patients with BRCA-positive and BRCA-negative breast cancer. J Clin Oncol. 2008;26:4282–8.
7. Mavaddat N, Barrowdale D, Andrulis IL, et al. Pathology of breast and ovarian cancers among BRCA1 and BRCA2 mutation carriers: results from the Consortium of Investigators of Modifiers of BRCA1/2 (CIMBA). Cancer Epidemiol Biomarkers Prev. 2012;21:134–47.
8. Tun NM, Villani G, Ong K, et al. Risk of having BRCA1 mutation in high-risk women with triple-negative breast cancer: a meta-analysis. Clin Genet. 2014;85:43–8.
9. Young SR, Pilarski RT, Donenberg T, et al. The prevalence of BRCA1 mutations among young women with triple-negative breast cancer. BMC Cancer. 2009;9:86.

10. Evans DG, Howell A, Ward D, et al. Prevalence of BRCA1 and BRCA2 mutations in triple negative breast cancer. J Med Genet. 2011;48:520–2.
11. Couch FJ, Hart SN, Sharma P, et al. Inherited mutations in 17 breast cancer susceptibility genes among a large triple-negative breast cancer cohort unselected for family history of breast cancer. J Clin Oncol. 2015;33:304–11.
12. Fostira F, Tsitlaidou M, Papadimitriou C, et al. Prevalence of BRCA1 mutations among 403 women with triple-negative breast cancer: implications for genetic screening selection criteria: a Hellenic Cooperative Oncology Group Study. Breast Cancer Res Treat. 2012;134:353–62.
13. Gonzalez-Angulo AM, Timms KM, Liu S, et al. Incidence and outcome of BRCA mutations in unselected patients with triple receptor-negative breast cancer. Clin Cancer Res. 2011;17:1082–9.
14. Rummel S, Varner E, Shriver CD, et al. Evaluation of BRCA1 mutations in an unselected patient population with triple-negative breast cancer. Breast Cancer Res Treat. 2013;137:119–25.
15. Greenup R, Buchanan A, Lorizio W, et al. Prevalence of BRCA mutations among women with triple-negative breast cancer (TNBC) in a genetic counseling cohort. Ann Surg Oncol. 2013;20:3254–8.
16. Struewing JP, Hartge P, Wacholder S, et al. The risk of cancer associated with specific mutations of BRCA1 and BRCA2 among Ashkenazi Jews. N Engl J Med. 1997;336:1401–8.
17. Comen E, Davids M, Kirchhoff T, et al. Relative contributions of BRCA1 and BRCA2 mutations to "triple-negative" breast cancer in Ashkenazi Women. Breast Cancer Res Treat. 2011;129:185–90.
18. Kurian AW, Fish K, Shema SJ, et al. Lifetime risks of specific breast cancer subtypes among women in four racial/ethnic groups. Breast Cancer Res. 2010;12:R99.
19. Huo D, Ikpatt F, Khramtsov A, et al. Population differences in breast cancer: survey in indigenous African women reveals over-representation of triple-negative breast cancer. J Clin Oncol. 2009;27:4515–21.
20. Fackenthal JD, Zhang J, Zhang B, et al. High prevalence of BRCA1 and BRCA2 mutations in unselected Nigerian breast cancer patients. Int J Cancer. 2012;131:1114–23.
21. Churpek JE, Walsh T, Zheng Y, et al. Inherited predisposition to breast cancer among African American women. Breast Cancer Res Treat. 2015;149:31–9.
22. Daly MB, Pilarski R, Axilbund JE, et al. Genetic/familial high-risk assessment: breast and ovarian, version 2.2015. J Natl Compr Canc Netw. 2016;14:153–62.
23. Masciari S, Dillon DA, Rath M, et al. Breast cancer phenotype in women with TP53 germline mutations: a Li-Fraumeni syndrome consortium effort. Breast Cancer Res Treat. 2012;133:1125–30.
24. Hwang SJ, Lozano G, Amos CI, et al. Germline p53 mutations in a cohort with childhood sarcoma: sex differences in cancer risk. Am J Hum Genet. 2003;72:975–83.
25. Figueiredo BC, Sandrini R, Zambetti GP, et al. Penetrance of adrenocortical tumours associated with the germline TP53 R337H mutation. J Med Genet. 2006;43:91–6.
26. Robson ME, Bradbury AR, Arun B, et al. American Society of Clinical Oncology Policy Statement update: genetic and genomic testing for cancer susceptibility. J Clin Oncol. 2015;33:3660–7.
27. Berliner JL, Fay AM, Cummings SA, et al. NSGC practice guideline: risk assessment and genetic counseling for hereditary breast and ovarian cancer. J Genet Couns. 2013;22:155–63.
28. Weitzel JN, Blazer KR, MacDonald DJ, et al. Genetics, genomics, and cancer risk assessment: state of the art and future directions in the era of personalized medicine. CA Cancer J Clin. 2011;61:327–59.
29. Tyrer J, Duffy SW, Cuzick J. A breast cancer prediction model incorporating familial and personal risk factors. Stat Med. 2004;23:1111–30.
30. Warner E, Plewes DB, Hill KA, et al. Surveillance of BRCA1 and BRCA2 mutation carriers with magnetic resonance imaging, ultrasound, mammography, and clinical breast examination. JAMA. 2004;292:1317–25.

31. Kriege M, Brekelmans CT, Boetes C, et al. Efficacy of MRI and mammography for breast-cancer screening in women with a familial or genetic predisposition. N Engl J Med. 2004;351:427–37.
32. Lehman CD, Lee JM, DeMartini WB, et al. Screening MRI in women with a personal history of breast cancer. J Natl Cancer Inst. 2016;108. pii: djv373.
33. Li X, You R, Wang X, et al. Effectiveness of prophylactic surgeries in BRCA1 or BRCA2 mutation carriers: a meta-analysis and systematic review. Clin Cancer Res. 2016;22:3971–81.
34. Evans DG, Gaarenstroom KN, Stirling D, et al. Screening for familial ovarian cancer: poor survival of BRCA1/2 related cancers. J Med Genet. 2009;46:593–7.
35. Rebbeck TR, Kauff ND, Domchek SM. Meta-analysis of risk reduction estimates associated with risk-reducing salpingo-oophorectomy in BRCA1 or BRCA2 mutation carriers. J Natl Cancer Inst. 2009;101:80–7.
36. Kauff ND, Domchek SM, Friebel TM, et al. Risk-reducing salpingo-oophorectomy for the prevention of BRCA1- and BRCA2-associated breast and gynecologic cancer: a multicenter, prospective study. J Clin Oncol. 2008;26:1331–7.
37. Irvin WJ Jr, Carey LA. What is triple-negative breast cancer? Eur J Cancer. 2008;44:2799–805.
38. Carey LA, Dees EC, Sawyer L, et al. The triple negative paradox: primary tumor chemosensitivity of breast cancer subtypes. Clin Cancer Res. 2007;13:2329–34.
39. Robson M, Im SA, Senkus E, et al. Olaparib for metastatic breast cancer in patients with a germline BRCA mutation. N Engl J Med. 2017;377:523–33.

Imaging of Triple-Negative Breast Cancer

4

Ann R. Mootz and Basak E. Dogan

Clinical Pearls
- Triple-negative breast cancers (TNBCs) identified in the general screening population are more likely to be interval cancers.
- The mammographic hallmark of TNBC is a mass, often with convex or "pushing" margins. Spiculations or irregular shape may be absent. Calcifications occur relatively rarely in TNBC.
- On ultrasound, TNBCs tend to exhibit round or oval shape, partially circumscribed margins, and parallel orientation to the chest wall, which are features that mimic a benign mass, cyst, or breast abscess.
- It is important to evaluate regional nodes with imaging to help identify clinically occult metastatic nodes early in the disease and appropriately route patients who may benefit from neoadjuvant chemotherapy (NAC).
- Dynamic contrast-enhanced (DCE)-MRI is more sensitive in detecting additional unsuspected disease in the breast than mammography and ultrasound, and its use can be considered in patients with TNBC, in whom the lack of targeted adjuvant endocrine therapies makes detection of true disease extent of critical importance for surgical management.
- DCE-MRI is more sensitive than mammography and ultrasound in evaluating the response to NAC, helps detect response sooner, and allows early and appropriate tailoring of NAC.

A.R. Mootz, MD (✉) • B.E. Dogan, MD, FSBI
Department of Diagnostic Radiology, The University of Texas Southwestern Medical Center, Dallas, TX, USA
e-mail: ann.mootz@utsouthwestern.edu; basak.dogan@utsouthwestern.edu

© Springer International Publishing AG 2018
A.R. Tan (ed.), *Triple-Negative Breast Cancer*,
https://doi.org/10.1007/978-3-319-69980-6_4

4.1   Introduction

Estrogen receptor (ER)-negative, progesterone receptor (PR)-negative, and human epidermal growth factor receptor 2 (HER2)-negative breast cancer, the so-called triple-negative breast cancer (TNBC), is a distinct breast cancer phenotype, often associated with young age, high histologic grade, a basal-like gene expression profile, suppressed *BRCA1* function, and poor prognosis [1, 2]. Imaging findings closely mirror that of clinical presentation and prognosis in TNBC, in that certain imaging features and patterns are overrepresented. We will present key imaging features characteristic of TNBC by mammography, ultrasound, dynamic contrast-enhanced (DCE) breast MRI, and positron emission mammography (PEM), focusing on the appropriate clinical application of each imaging technique, along with potential benefits or pitfalls.

Due to the aggressive biological behavior of these tumors, their rapid growth, and the fact that they can occur in younger women with dense breast tissue, TNBC is unlikely to be found with routine screening mammography alone. In fact, TNBCs identified in the general screening population are more likely to be an interval cancer, which is a cancer that becomes clinically evident between two routine screening mammograms [3].

Because TNBC is difficult to detect with screening mammography alone, patients with TNBC usually present with clinical findings. In a large series of TNBCs, an abnormal screening mammogram resulted in the diagnosis of TNBC in only 28.5% of patients. The remaining patients were diagnosed clinically. Clinical findings present at the time of diagnosis included a palpable mass (59.3% of patients), nipple discharge (1.7%), breast pain (5.4%), inverted nipple (0.7%), and breast swelling (1.4%) [4].

While mammography may have a limited role in imaging TNBC, ultrasound is more useful in detecting, characterizing, staging, and monitoring response to chemotherapy. Unlike other breast cancer subtypes in which the utilization of whole-breast ultrasound and MRI to determine disease extent is controversial, in TNBC, given the lack of targeted endocrine therapy to be used in the adjuvant setting, the poor prognosis, and the potential for untreated reservoir sites to contribute to distant recurrence, identifying full disease extent is critical.

Ultrasound provides a cost-effective means of determining the extent of regional lymph node disease. Unlike the ER- and HER2-positive breast cancer subtypes, there appears to be an uncoupling of the usual positive association between tumor size, lymph node status, and overall survival (OS) in patients with TNBC [5, 6]. Even patients with tumors less than 1–2 cm in size are likely to be node positive at the time of diagnosis. In Dent's series, 55% of patients with tumors less than 1.0 cm in size had at least one positive lymph node [6]. Thus, patients with seemingly early-stage breast cancer may already have locoregional or distant metastases. Parallel to this finding, the survival rates of TNBC patients are significantly decreased compared to patients with ER- and HER2-positive tumors in the first

3 years after treatment, suggesting that the more frequent occurrence of early lymph node metastasis in TNBC may play a significant role in determining disease prognosis.

4.2 Key Mammographic Features of Triple-Negative Breast Cancer

Parallel to having a typical demographic pattern and clinical presentation, imaging findings in the TNBC phenotype have also been shown to be characteristic. The mammographic hallmark of TNBC is a mass, often with convex or "pushing" margins [7]. The margins of the mass may be partially circumscribed [8]. TNBC oftentimes lacks the mammographic features typically associated with malignancy such as an irregular mass shape and spiculations, which are seen more commonly in ER-positive and HER2-positive tumors [9]. The combination of a partially circumscribed mass having convex and partially circumscribed margins can mimic a benign process such as a fibroadenoma. This relatively "benign" appearance of TNBC can lead to a delay in the diagnosis, especially in younger women in whom complicated cysts or palpable fibroadenomas are prevalent.

Conversely, calcifications occur much less frequently in TNBC (15%) compared to ER-positive (61%) and HER2-positive (67%) cancers ($P < 0.0001$) [1]. The lack of calcifications is an important finding that differentiates these cancers from other molecular subtypes, especially because this feature has been shown to correlate to the absence of ductal carcinoma in situ (DCIS) histopathologically. Based on the absence of calcifications and concomitant DCIS in TNBC, investigators have suggested that rapid carcinogenesis in TNBC leads directly to invasive cancer, bypassing the precancerous or in situ phase of carcinoma [1].

The mammographic features of a benign-appearing mass and the absence of calcifications seen in TNBC have also been described in patients with familial breast cancer [10, 11]. Warner noted that cancers in *BRCA1* mutation carriers tended to be more cellular with round and "pushing" margins on mammography rather than irregular in shape. DCIS without invasion, presenting solely as calcifications on a mammogram, did not occur in any of the *BRCA1* mutation carriers in her series. Patients with *BRCA2* mutations exhibited the mammographic features more typically associated with ER- and HER2-positive breast cancer, such as an irregular mass shape and calcifications on the mammogram. Indeed, DCIS without invasion was only seen in *BRCA2* mutation carriers.

While there are consistent, distinguishing mammographic features that help use imaging as a surrogate marker to distinguish TNBC from other breast cancer subtypes, certain subgroups of TNBC deviate from this characteristic imaging phenotype. More recent analysis of the mammographic, sonographic, and MRI features in a distinct subgroup of TNBC that express androgen receptors (AR) shows that AR-positive TNBCs tend to have the mammographic features more commonly seen in ER and HER2 molecular subtypes. The presence of mammographic calcifications with or without a mass, masses with irregular shape or spiculated margins, and non-mass enhancement on MRI were significantly associated with AR-positive TNBC [12]. Compared to AR-negative TNBC, AR-positive TNBCs are histopathologically more likely to have a DCIS component (90.9% versus 59.8%; $P < 0.001$) [12] and are therefore more frequently associated with mammographic calcifications and non-mass enhancement on MRI [12].

4.3   Ultrasound Findings of Triple-Negative Breast Cancer

Most TNBCs present as a mass on ultrasound. Similar to that of mammography, TNBCs may exhibit ultrasound features that favor a benign process, including round or oval shape, partially circumscribed margins, or parallel orientation to the chest wall. The masses are usually hypoechoic and oftentimes markedly hypoechoic ($P < 0.0001$) [13], a finding that may mimic a benign cyst or breast abscess. Posterior acoustic enhancement, an ultrasound feature typically encountered in benign cysts or abscesses as a result of rapid sound transmission through the fluid portion of the imaged tissue, occurs more commonly in TNBC than in the other breast cancer subtypes (36.4% versus 13.0%) [14]. Posterior acoustic enhancement is likely an imaging manifestation of internal tumor necrosis that increases the "nonsolid" tumor content and is a common feature in TNBC histopathologically, independent of tumor size. A combination of predominantly benign margin features and internal or posterior acoustic signs signaling cystic contents may lead to radiologists falsely classifying a TNBC as a benign process. Therefore, any newly palpable mass in a young woman which is not a simple cyst should be subjected to needle biopsy or short-term follow-up to mitigate a possible delay in TNBC diagnosis (Fig. 4.1a, b, and c).

The usual sonographic features associated with malignancy, such as an irregular mass shape, occur much less frequently in TNBC (Fig. 4.1c). Posterior acoustical shadowing and an echogenic halo also occur much less frequently [13, 14].

Fig. 4.1 A 42-year-old African-American woman presenting with interval triple-negative breast cancer. (**a**) A routine yearly craniocaudal (CC) screening mammogram is normal. The clip (arrow) is related to a prior benign biopsy. (**b**) Four months later, the patient developed a palpable mass in the left breast. On the CC mammogram, a 1.5 cm partially circumscribed mass (orange arrow) is present corresponding to the palpable mass. (**c**) Transverse gray-scale ultrasound of the palpable mass shows a markedly hypoechoic mass with posterior acoustic enhancement (arrowheads). Because of its relatively benign appearance, ultrasound-guided aspiration (not shown) was attempted but was unsuccessful and returned blood. Ultrasound-guided core needle biopsy of the mass was TNBC. (**d**) Axillary ultrasound demonstrated a single enlarged lymph node measuring 4.0 cm with marked cortical thickening (arrow). (**e**) Ultrasound-guided core needle biopsy was performed of the lymph node, and a clip (arrow) was placed within the node. The biopsy was positive for metastatic TNBC from the breast primary tumor. (**f**) An early-phase DCE-MRI subtraction axial image shows an enhancing mass (red arrow) with mammographically and sonographically occult multifocal disease (orange arrow). (**g**) The patient received six cycles of NAC. At the time of bilateral mastectomy and SLNB, the single metastatic lymph node was identified as containing the clip (arrow) placed at the time of the ultrasound-guided biopsy. This node was positive for micrometastatic disease

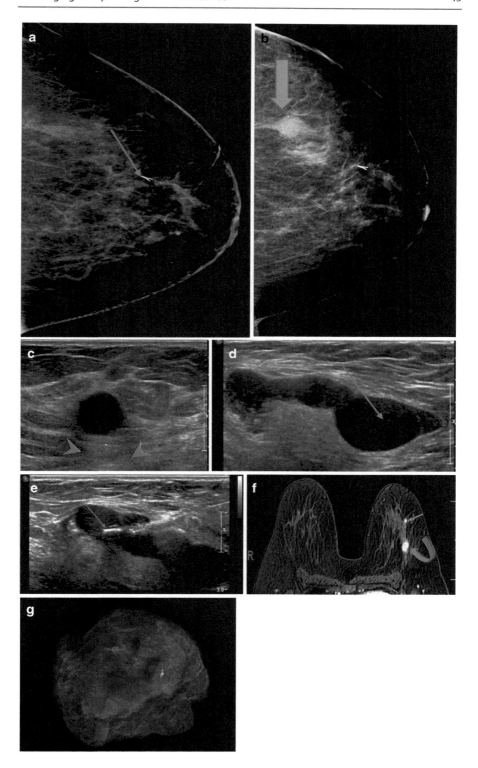

4.4   Role of Ultrasound in Evaluating Regional Lymph Node Basins

While breast cancer subtypes have become essential to guide systemic therapy, regional lymph node status remains important to decide the sequence, type, and extent of systemic therapy [6]. Because of the high frequency of metastatic lymphadenopathy at the time of diagnosis, thorough evaluation of all regional lymph node basins is critical to accurately determine the stage of disease even in small TNBCs (Fig. 4.1d). Identifying clinically occult lymph node metastases on ultrasound may lead to important changes in management of the patient, resulting in the conversion of initially planned up-front surgery to neoadjuvant chemotherapy or boosting nodal adjuvant radiotherapy.

The routine use of ultrasound in the evaluation of the axillary, infraclavicular, supraclavicular, and internal mammary lymph node chains has been previously described in detail [15]. Ultrasound is a reliable method of evaluating the regional nodal basins, and its use may obviate the need for costlier imaging modalities such as MRI and fluorine-18 fluorodeoxyglucose (FDG) positron emission tomography (^{18}F FDG-PET). The routine use of ultrasound in evaluation of all regional lymph node basins increases the rate of positive regional nodal disease for patients with TNBC, beyond the clinical stage determined by physical examination and mammography alone, in roughly 20% of patients [4]. Importantly, ultrasound leads to significant management changes in these patients. Higher proportions of TNBC patients were treated with neoadjuvant chemotherapy (NAC) (91.9% versus 51.2%, $P < 0.0001$), axillary lymph node dissection (91.1% versus 34.5%, $P < 0.0001$), and adjuvant radiotherapy to the regional nodal basins (88.2% versus 29.2%, $P < 0.001$) compared to patients whose disease was not upstaged [4]. The axillary response rates to neoadjuvant chemotherapy differ significantly by tumor subtype with complete eradication of disease seen in 38.2% of patients with TNBC, in 45.4% of HER2-positive tumors, but in only 11.4% of ER-positive tumors ($P < 0.0001$) [16]. Because a complete response to therapy may cause positive lymph nodes to go undiagnosed, knowing the status of all regional lymph node basins prior to beginning treatment is important for surgical planning as well as determining the need for adjuvant radiotherapy. Therefore, ultrasound of the regional nodes is an important tool that leads to the earlier discovery of unsuspected nodal metastasis, often leading to more aggressive therapy in the management of TNBC patients.

In patients with sonographically suspicious axillary lymph nodes, ultrasound-guided fine needle aspiration biopsy (FNAB) or core biopsy should be performed to confirm the presence of metastatic disease. It is important to mark the "index" lymph node that was biopsied with a clip to ensure its removal at the time of axillary lymph node dissection (Fig. 4.1e). This is especially important for TNBC patients who are more likely to be treated with preoperative NAC, since the American College of Surgeons Oncology Group (ACOSOG) Z1071 trial showed that sentinel lymph node biopsy (SLNB) is not sufficiently predictive of residual axillary metastatic disease [17]. SLNB may miss the residual metastatic node in 12% of patients, rendering SLNB unreliable as a stand-alone diagnostic tool after NAC. However, marking the index axillary node with a clip, localizing it preoperatively, and removing it at the time of SLNB significantly decreases the false negative rate to 2% or less and may allow patients with preoperative axillary complete response to NAC avoid the morbidity of a full axillary lymph node dissection (Fig. 4.1g) [18].

Routine evaluation of the internal mammary (IM) lymph nodal basins with ultrasound is also important particularly since IM lymph nodes are not accessible to physical examination. Although ultrasound detected abnormal IM lymph nodes in only 10% of breast cancer patients of all subtypes, patients with younger age ($P < 0.0001$), with tumors greater than 5 cm in size ($P < 0.001$), of high histologic grade ($P < 0.0001$), triple-negative subtype ($P < 0.001$), and associated with axillary ($P < 0.0001$), infraclavicular ($P < 0.0001$), or supraclavicular ($P < 0.0001$) lymphadenopathy were significantly more likely to have positive IM lymph nodes at ultrasound [19]. IM ultrasound resulted in a nodal stage change in 69% of these patients. The presence of unsuspected IM disease in patients thought to have early Stage or II disease resulted in significant upstaging of the patient's disease to Stage III. This upstaging of disease had important clinical and prognostic implications, resulting in changes in surgical management and adjuvant radiotherapy.

4.5 Dynamic Contrast-Enhanced Magnetic Resonance Imaging of Triple-Negative Breast Cancer

4.5.1 DCE-MRI Features of Triple-Negative Breast Cancer

Similar to mammography and ultrasound, MRI findings in TNBC have consistently been found to be distinctive compared to non-TNBC. TNBC most commonly appears as a mass on DCE-MRI in up to 95% of cases, often with convex borders [20]. The average tumor size of TNBC is significantly larger on MRI than ER- and HER2-positive tumors, ranging in size from 4 to 10 cm in one series with 79% of patients presenting at stage T2 or above [21]. The masses are most often unifocal. Intratumoral high or very high signal intensity on T2-weighted images is significantly associated with TNBC and is key to identifying TNBC on imaging [20]. This high signal intensity on T2-weighted images corresponds to the intratumoral necrosis that is present pathologically [22].

The predominant pattern of enhancement seen in TNBC is rim enhancement as reported across multiple series of patients [2, 7, 22–26]. This is in keeping with the pattern of rim enhancement that is seen in invasive cancers of higher histologic grade, larger size, and associated with a higher incidence of axillary metastasis [27]. Indeed, rim enhancement may be the most useful MR finding in identifying TNBC [28]. Internal enhancing septations were observed in 30% of cases reported by Dogan et al. [7].

TNBC demonstrates the kinetic curves typically associated with malignancy, with rapid washin and washout of contrast [21, 22, 24]. However, up to 50% of TNBC cases may demonstrate a persistent enhancement pattern, which is more frequently associated with benign enhancing processes [22].

Table 4.1 Summary meta-analysis of reported mammographic, sonographic, and MRI imaging feature statistics in 863 patients with triple-negative breast cancer [1, 7, 9, 13, 14, 22, 24, 47]

American College of Radiology© BIRADS feature[a]	Mean (%)	Median (%)	Range %
Mammography BIRADS features (N = 631)[b]			
Mass only	377 (59.4)	334 (53)	49–62
Mass with associated calcifications	91 (14.6)	95 (15)	5–21
Focal asymmetry	77 (12.2)	58 (9)	9–22
Calcifications only	48 (7.6)	44 (7)	0–13
Architectural distortion	38 (6)	16 (2.5)	0–5
Total mammography features	631 (100)		
Ultrasound BIRADS features (N = 464)			
Mass	274 (71)	288 (79)	40–92
Architectural distortion	37 (8)	37 (8)	2–14
No lesions	40 (8.6)	28 (6)	6–20
Other	116 (12)	111 (7)	0–20
Total ultrasound features	464 (100)		
Mass features (N = 278)			
Hypoechoic or markedly hypoechoic	241 (86.7)	245 (87)	80–90
[c]Posterior acoustic enhancement	125 (45)	125 (45)	41–49
MRI BIRADS features (N = 243)			
Mass-like enhancement	199 (82)	190 (78)	75–95
Non-mass-like enhancement	32 (13)	33 (13.5)	22–60
Enhancement time-intensity kinetics			
Washout kinetics (type 3)	162 (66.7)	146 (60)	60–90
Other kinetics (plateau or progressive types)	81 (33.3)	97 (40)	9–50

[a]*ACR BI-RADS® Atlas, Breast Imaging Reporting and Data System. Reston, VA, American College of Radiology; 2013*
[b]Mammography was negative in median of 88 (14%) patients (range 9–18%), reported in two series
[c]See Fig. 4.1 for the depiction of posterior acoustic enhancement

A summary of the imaging features of TNBC on mammography, ultrasound, and MRI across multiple single institution studies is provided in Table 4.1.

4.5.2 Role of DCE-MRI in Preoperative Staging of Triple-Negative Breast Cancer

The routine use of MRI in the preoperative staging of breast cancer remains controversial. MRI is more sensitive than mammography or ultrasound in the measurement of tumor size and in the detection of multifocal, multicentric, or contralateral disease in the breast. Despite these advantages, the widespread use of routine preoperative MRI has not been shown to reduce the rates of surgical re-excision, and, at the same time, its use has increased the rate of mastectomy [29, 30]. Additionally, a positive effect of preoperative MRI on long-term survival has not been shown [31]. A likely explanation of why MRI's higher sensitivity did not translate into improved surgical outcomes is that, although MRI-detected additional disease is implicated by the radiologist, not all patients have access to or are submitted to MRI-guided percutaneous needle biopsy to confirm true disease extent. Therefore, a large majority of patients who have preoperative MRI either prefer to have mastectomy based on perceived large disease extent or they undergo breast-conserving therapy (segmental mastectomy or lumpectomy) in an attempt to remove unmarked and radiographically occult additional sites of disease that are difficult to identify, document, or assess margin status intraoperatively by the surgeon. However, the potential benefit of preoperative MRI in patients with a high-risk molecular subtype such as TNBC is still under investigation.

Although preoperative DCE-MRI was more likely to depict multifocal or multicentric disease in ER and HER2 molecular subtypes (53.3% and 65.4% of cases), Grimm reported an incidence of multifocal and multicentric disease in 27% of TNBC [32]. This is similar to the rate of multifocal disease in the two series of TNBC reported by Dogan and Chen [7, 21] (Fig. 4.1f). The presence of this unsuspected additional disease had important clinical implications, resulting in a change in the surgical plan in 10% of patients in a large series of TNBCs reported by Lee [33].

One of the arguments against the routine use of preoperative MRI for surgical planning in early breast cancer patients who are eligible to undergo breast-conserving surgery is the significant added benefit of adjuvant chemotherapy and radiotherapy which likely treats mammographically and clinically undetected additional foci of disease. However, identifying occult multifocal and multicentric disease in TNBC is likely more prognostically relevant than in the ER-positive and HER2-positive molecular subtypes because adjuvant endocrine therapy is not available to treat TNBC patients. In an analysis of the prognostic significance of multifocal or multicentric disease identified on MRI among the various breast cancer subtypes [34], the prognostic significance of multifocal or multicentric disease on metastasis-free survival was seen only in the TNBC subtype, suggesting that it is these additional foci of disease that contribute to distant metastasis. The presence of multifocal and multicentric disease was associated with an increased incidence of subsequent distant metastasis and death only when the cancers were the triple-negative subtype. Therefore, all multifocal and multicentric disease found on MRI in TNBC patients should be considered clinically significant [34].

The failure of TNBC patients to undergo preoperative MRI is significantly associated with breast cancer recurrence, even in patients with early-stage disease. In a large series of patients undergoing preoperative MRI, the overall 10-year risk of ipsilateral breast cancer recurrence across all breast cancer subtypes was 3.6% [35]. Recurrence of breast cancer in the same breast was greatest in a high-risk group that included TNBC and HER2-positive tumors compared with the other tumor subtypes (9.8% vs. 1.7%, $P < 0.001$). In the patients with TNBC and HER2-positive tumors who did *not* undergo preoperative MRI, the ipsilateral breast cancer recurrence rate was even higher (11.8%) compared to the remainder of tumor subtypes (1.8%). Therefore, we could likely conclude that in TNBC patients, in whom mammographically dense breasts may mask MRI-detectable additional invasive TNBC foci, preoperative MRI should be considered before attempting breast-conserving therapy.

4.5.3   Role of DCE-MRI in Monitoring Response to Neoadjuvant Chemotherapy

Achieving a complete pathologic response (pCR) following NAC is associated with recurrence-free (RF) and overall survival (OS) benefits. Furthermore, achieving pCR after NAC differs among breast cancer subtypes. TNBCs have higher rates of pCR than ER-positive tumors (22% versus 11%), and patients with TNBC who demonstrate pCR have OS rates approaching that of the non-TNBC subtypes [36]. Furthermore, patients with residual disease following NAC have worse overall survival if they have TNBC compared to non-TNBC subtypes, particularly in the first 3 years after diagnosis [36].

The sensitivity of MRI in the detection of residual disease following NAC is much higher compared to mammography, ultrasound, and clinical examination [28, 37–40]. Because TNBC most often occurs as a single mass, the presence of decreasing mass size on MRI makes MRI well suited to detecting a response to therapy in this group of patients. ER-positive tumors often have non-mass enhancement making MRI less accurate in determining response to NAC than the TNBC and HER2-positive subgroups. Changes at MRI *during* NAC correlated well with pCR for TNBC and HER2-positive breast cancer but not for ER-positive tumors [41]. Monitoring the response to chemotherapy is important in patient management decisions, perhaps allowing for a change in therapy or sparing the patient the side effects of ineffective therapy.

4.6   Long-Term Follow-Up of Patients with Triple-Negative Breast Cancer

The patterns of recurrence in patients with TNBC are both qualitatively and quantitatively different than the other breast cancer subtypes [6]. Patients with TNBC are distinct from the ER- and HER-positive subtypes in that they have a higher incidence of metastasis to visceral organs including the brain, liver, and lung, early in the course of disease. Bone metastasis is more common in ER-positive tumors. The higher incidence of visceral metastasis may help explain why patients with TNBC have higher rates of recurrence and death compared to the other breast cancer subtypes only within the first 3 years following diagnosis, decreasing rapidly thereafter [6]. Unlike patients with the other breast cancer subtypes, recurrence after 8 years is uncommon indicating that a "cure" may be possible in some patients [42].

Given the high rate of visceral metastasis, patients with TNBC may require closer surveillance in the first 3 years following diagnosis. [18]F FDG-PET is of limited usefulness in the evaluation of ER- and HER2-positive breast cancers because of the low uptake of radiotracer into the primary tumor. TNBC has a much greater avidity for FDG because of an increase in glycolysis in this tumor subtype, with sensitivities approaching 100% in detecting the primary tumor [43]. [18]F FDG-PET is also sensitive in the detection of extra-axillary nodal disease and in detecting distant metastasis. National Comprehensive Cancer Network (NCCN) guidelines recommend reserving ^{18}F FDG-PET for patients presenting with Stage III breast cancer. However, a recent study of ^{18}F FDG-PET in TNBC patients thought to be Stage I or II found unexpected extra-axillary nodal disease or distant metastases in 15% of patients [44]. Unsuspected synchronous malignances outside the breast were also found in 5% of patients. This upstaging of disease had important implications for patient management, with the presence of distant metastasis resulting in palliative rather than surgical care.

Positron emission mammography (PEM) may be a useful adjunct in patients already undergoing ^{18}F FDG-PET. PEM has been shown to detect malignancies not seen with mammography and ultrasound with an overall sensitivity of 90% [45]. Additionally, the use of views similar to the routine views obtained with mammography has certain advantages in interpretation. However, the need for the patient to be fasting and the long time period required to obtain an image (10 min per view) limit its routine use. It may, however, be used in patients unable to undergo MRI as its sensitivity in detecting multiple foci of disease approaches that of MRI. Additionally, the positive predictive value (ppv) of PEM-detected biopsies (66%) is much higher than MRI (53%) [46]. The capacity to do PEM-guided biopsy is limited at the present time. If a lesion is detected only by PEM, in some instances, second-look ultrasound has been used successfully to guide percutaneous needle biopsy for lesions detected only with PEM.

4.7 Summary

TNBC is a breast cancer subtype with a distinctive clinical presentation and phenotypic expression on imaging. TNBC most often presents mammographically as a mass, often with benign-appearing features on ultrasound, which may lead to incorrect interpretation of this highly aggressive tumor subtype as benign. Ultrasound is a widely available and cost-effective imaging modality used for evaluation of all regional lymph node basins which is particularly important in patients with TNBC given the high rate of axillary metastases present at the time of diagnosis. Ultrasound may also be used to evaluate response to NAC in patients unable to undergo MRI. DCE-MRI is very sensitive in the detection of multifocal and multicentric disease in the breast, which, given the lack of targeted adjuvant therapies for TNBC, is critical in determining appropriate surgical management. DCE-MRI is also more sensitive than mammography and ultrasound in assessing for pCR following NAC. Because routine screening with mammography alone is unlikely to detect TNBC, novel methods for earlier detection of this highly aggressive tumor subtype are needed if the disease is to be detected before clinical symptoms develop and distant metastasis may have already occurred.

References

 1. Yang WT, Dryden M, Broglio K, Gilcrease M, Dawood S, Dempsey PJ, et al. Mammographic features of triple receptor-negative primary breast cancers in young premenopausal women. Breast Cancer Res Treat. 2008;111(3):405–10.
 2. Boisserie-Lacroix M, MacGrogan G, Debled M, Ferron S, Asad-Syed M, McKelvie-Sebileau P, et al. Triple-negative breast cancers: associations between imaging and pathological findings for triple-negative tumors compared with hormone receptor-positive/human epidermal growth factor receptor-2-negative breast cancers. Oncologist. 2013;18(7):802–11.
 3. Collett K, Stefansson IM, Eide J, Braaten A, Wang H, Eide GE, et al. A basal epithelial phenotype is more frequent in interval breast cancers compared with screen detected tumors. Cancer Epidemiol Biomark Prev. 2005;14(5):1108–12.
 4. Shaitelman SF, Tereffe W, Dogan BE, Hess KR, Caudle AS, Valero V, et al. Role of ultrasonography of regional nodal basins in staging triple-negative breast cancer and implications for local-regional treatment. Int J Radiat Oncol Biol Phys. 2015;93(1):102–10.
 5. Foulkes WD, Metcalfe K, Hanna W, Lynch HT, Ghadirian P, Tung N, et al. Disruption of the expected positive correlation between breast tumor size and lymph node status in BRCA1-related breast carcinoma. Cancer. 2003;98(8):1569–77.
 6. Dent R, Trudeau M, Pritchard KI, Hanna WM, Kahn HK, Sawka CA, et al. Triple-negative breast cancer: clinical features and patterns of recurrence. Clin Cancer Res. 2007;13(15 Pt 1):4429–34.
 7. Dogan BE, Gonzalez-Angulo AM, Gilcrease M, Dryden MJ, Yang WT. Multimodality imaging of triple receptor-negative tumors with mammography, ultrasound, and MRI. AJR Am J Roentgenol. 2010;194(4):1160–6.
 8. Dogan BE, Turnbull LW. Imaging of triple-negative breast cancer. Ann Oncol. 2012;23(Suppl 6):vi23–9.
 9. Wang Y, Ikeda DM, Narasimhan B, Longacre TA, Bleicher RJ, Pal S, et al. Estrogen receptor-negative invasive breast cancer: imaging features of tumors with and without human epidermal growth factor receptor type 2 overexpression. Radiology. 2008;246(2):367–75.
10. Warner E, Plewes DB, Hill KA, Causer PA, Zubovits JT, Jong RA, et al. Surveillance of BRCA1 and BRCA2 mutation carriers with magnetic resonance imaging, ultrasound, mammography, and clinical breast examination. JAMA. 2004;292(11):1317–25.
11. Schrading S, Kuhl CK. Mammographic, US, and MR imaging phenotypes of familial breast cancer. Radiology. 2008;246(1):58–70.
12. Bae MS, Park SY, Song SE, Kim WH, Lee SH, Han W, et al. Heterogeneity of triple-negative breast cancer: mammographic, US, and MR imaging features according to androgen receptor expression. Eur Radiol. 2015;25(2):419–27.
13. Ko ES, Lee BH, Kim HA, Noh WC, Kim MS, Lee SA. Triple-negative breast cancer: correlation between imaging and pathological findings. Eur Radiol. 2010;20(5):1111–7.
14. Wojcinski S, Soliman AA, Schmidt J, Makowski L, Degenhardt F, Hillemanns P. Sonographic features of triple-negative and non-triple-negative breast cancer. J Ultrasound Med. 2012;31(10):1531–41.
15. Fornage BD. Local and regional staging of invasive breast cancer with sonography: 25 years of practice at MD Anderson Cancer Center. Oncologist. 2014;19(1):5–15.
16. Boughey JC, McCall LM, Ballman KV, Mittendorf EA, Ahrendt GM, Wilke LG, et al. Tumor biology correlates with rates of breast-conserving surgery and pathologic complete response after neoadjuvant chemotherapy for breast cancer: findings from the ACOSOG Z1071 (alliance) prospective multicenter clinical trial. Ann Surg. 2014;260(4):608–14; discussion 14–6.
17. Boughey JC, Suman VJ, Mittendorf EA, Ahrendt GM, Wilke LG, Taback B, et al. Sentinel lymph node surgery after neoadjuvant chemotherapy in patients with node-positive breast cancer: the ACOSOG Z1071 (alliance) clinical trial. JAMA. 2013;310(14):1455–61.
18. Caudle AS, Yang WT, Krishnamurthy S, Mittendorf EA, Black DM, Gilcrease MZ, et al. Improved axillary evaluation following neoadjuvant therapy for patients with node-positive

breast cancer using selective evaluation of clipped nodes: implementation of targeted axillary dissection. J Clin Oncol. 2016;34(10):1072–8.

19. Dogan BE, Dryden MJ, Wei W, Fornage BD, Buchholz TA, Smith B, et al. Sonography and sonographically guided needle biopsy of internal mammary nodes in staging of patients with breast cancer. AJR Am J Roentgenol. 2015;205(4):905–11.

20. Uematsu T. MR imaging of triple-negative breast cancer. Breast Cancer. 2011;18(3):161–4.

21. Chen JH, Agrawal G, Feig B, Baek HM, Carpenter PM, Mehta RS, et al. Triple-negative breast cancer: MRI features in 29 patients. Ann Oncol. 2007;18(12):2042–3.

22. Uematsu T, Kasami M, Yuen S. Triple-negative breast cancer: correlation between MR imaging and pathologic findings. Radiology. 2009;250(3):638–47.

23. Youk JH, Son EJ, Chung J, Kim JA, Kim EK. Triple-negative invasive breast cancer on dynamic contrast-enhanced and diffusion-weighted MR imaging: comparison with other breast cancer subtypes. Eur Radiol. 2012;22(8):1724–34.

24. Sung JS, Jochelson MS, Brennan S, Joo S, Wen YH, Moskowitz C, et al. MR imaging features of triple-negative breast cancers. Breast J. 2013;19(6):643–9.

25. Costantini M, Belli P, Distefano D, Bufi E, Matteo MD, Rinaldi P, et al. Magnetic resonance imaging features in triple-negative breast cancer: comparison with luminal and HER2-overexpressing tumors. Clin Breast Cancer. 2012;12(5):331–9.

26. Fraguell MV, Criville MS, Ferrari JDR, Navarro FJA, Portulas ED, Roquerols JP, et al. Triple-negative breast carcinoma: heterogeneity in immunophenotypes and pharmacokinetic behavior. Radiologia. 2016;58(1):55–63.

27. Jinguji M, Kajiya Y, Kamimura K, Nakajo M, Sagara Y, Takahama T, et al. Rim enhancement of breast cancers on contrast-enhanced MR imaging: relationship with prognostic factors. Breast Cancer. 2006;13(1):64–73.

28. Li J, Han X. Research and progress in magnetic resonance imaging of triple-negative breast cancer. Magn Reson Imaging. 2014;32(4):392–6.

29. Turnbull L, Brown S, Harvey I, Olivier C, Drew P, Napp V, et al. Comparative effectiveness of MRI in breast cancer (COMICE) trial: a randomised controlled trial. Lancet. 2010;375(9714):563–71.

30. Houssami N, Turner R, Morrow M. Preoperative magnetic resonance imaging in breast cancer meta-analysis of surgical outcomes. Ann Surg. 2013;257(2):249–55.

31. Houssami N, Turner R, Macaskill P, Turnbull LW, McCready DR, Tuttle TM, et al. An individual person data meta-analysis of preoperative magnetic resonance imaging and breast cancer recurrence. J Clin Oncol. 2014;32(5):392–401.

32. Grimm LJ, Johnson KS, Marcom PK, Baker JA, Soo MS. Can breast cancer molecular subtype help to select patients for preoperative MR imaging? Radiology. 2015;274(2):352–8.

33. Lee J, Jung JH, Kim WW, Hwang SO, Kim HJ, Park JY, et al. The role of preoperative breast magnetic resonance (MR) imaging for surgical decision in patients with triple-negative breast cancer. J Surg Oncol. 2016;113(1):12–6.

34. Moon HG, Han W, Kim JY, Kim SJ, Yoon JH, SJ O, et al. Effect of multiple invasive foci on breast cancer outcomes according to the molecular subtypes: a report from the Korean Breast Cancer Society. Ann Oncol. 2013;24(9):2298–304.

35. Gervais MK, Maki E, Schiller DE, Crystal P, McCready DR. Preoperative MRI of the breast and ipsilateral breast tumor recurrence: long-term follow up. J Surg Oncol. 2017;115:231.

36. Liedtke C, Mazouni C, Hess KR, Andre F, Tordai A, Mejia JA, et al. Response to neoadjuvant therapy and long-term survival in patients with triple-negative breast cancer. J Clin Oncol. 2008;26(8):1275–81.

37. Nakahara H, Yasuda Y, Machida E, Maeda Y, Furusawa H, Komaki K, et al. MR and US imaging for breast cancer patients who underwent conservation surgery after neoadjuvant chemotherapy: comparison of triple negative breast cancer and other intrinsic subtypes. Breast Cancer. 2011;18(3):152–60.

38. Partridge SC, Gibbs JE, Lu Y, Esserman LJ, Sudilovsky D, Hylton NM. Accuracy of MR imaging for revealing residual breast cancer in patients who have undergone neoadjuvant chemotherapy. AJR Am J Roentgenol. 2002;179(5):1193–9.

39. Yeh E, Slanetz P, Kopans DB, Rafferty E, Georgian-Smith D, Moy L, et al. Prospective comparison of mammography, sonography, and MRI in patients undergoing neoadjuvant chemotherapy for palpable breast cancer. AJR Am J Roentgenol. 2005;184(3):868–77.
40. Hylton NM, Blume JD, Bernreuter WK, Pisano ED, Rosen MA, Morris EA, et al. Locally advanced breast cancer: MR imaging for prediction of response to neoadjuvant chemotherapy—results from ACRIN 6657/I-SPY TRIAL. Radiology. 2012;263(3):663–72.
41. Loo CE, Straver ME, Rodenhuis S, Muller SH, Wesseling J, Vrancken Peeters MJ, et al. Magnetic resonance imaging response monitoring of breast cancer during neoadjuvant chemotherapy: relevance of breast cancer subtype. J Clin Oncol. 2011;29(6):660–6.
42. Foulkes WD, Smith IE, Reis-Filho JS. Triple-negative breast cancer. N Engl J Med. 2010;363(20):1938–48.
43. Basu S, Chen W, Tchou J, Mavi A, Cermik T, Czerniecki B, et al. Comparison of triple-negative and estrogen receptor-positive/progesterone receptor-positive/HER2-negative breast carcinoma using quantitative fluorine-18 fluorodeoxyglucose/positron emission tomography imaging parameters: a potentially useful method for disease characterization. Cancer. 2008;112(5):995–1000.
44. Ulaner GA, Castillo R, Goldman DA, Wills J, Riedl CC, Pinker-Domenig K, et al. (18)F-FDG-PET/CT for systemic staging of newly diagnosed triple-negative breast cancer. Eur J Nucl Med Mol Imaging. 2016;43(11):1937–44.
45. Berg WA, Weinberg IN, Narayanan D, Lobrano ME, Ross E, Amodei L, et al. High-resolution fluorodeoxyglucose positron emission tomography with compression ("positron emission mammography") is highly accurate in depicting primary breast cancer. Breast J. 2006;12(4):309–23.
46. Berg WA, Madsen KS, Schilling K, Tartar M, Pisano ED, Larsen LH, et al. Breast cancer: comparative effectiveness of positron emission mammography and MR imaging in presurgical planning for the ipsilateral breast. Radiology. 2011;258(1):59–72.
47. Kojima Y, Tsunoda H. Mammography and ultrasound features of triple-negative breast cancer. Breast Cancer. 2011;18(3):146–51.

Surgical Management of Triple-Negative Breast Cancer

5

Ali Amro and Lisa A. Newman

Clinical Pearls
- Breast-conserving surgery is safe in triple-negative breast cancer (TNBC) patients as the increased risk of distant metastatic failure is not mitigated by mastectomy.
- In TNBC patients undergoing mastectomy, immediate reconstruction is safe.
- The management of the axilla and the prognostic value of nodal metastases in TNBC patients are similar to non-TNBC patients; this applies to lymphatic mapping and sentinel lymph node biopsy.
- Neoadjuvant chemotherapy as a treatment approach in TNBC can improve lumpectomy eligibility as well as downstage the axilla, thereby making axillary lymph node dissection less likely.

5.1 Introduction

Invasive cancers of the breast that are negative for the estrogen receptor (ER), the progesterone receptor (PR), and the human epidermal growth factor receptor type 2 (HER2) are commonly referred to as triple-negative breast cancer (TNBC). This category of breast cancer actually comprises a diverse spectrum of tumors, with some such as secretory and adenoid cystic carcinoma associated with a relatively favorable prognosis [1]. Approximately 80% of TNBCs belong to the biologically aggressive basal breast cancer subtype defined by gene expression profiling [2].

A. Amro, MD
Henry Ford Health System, Detroit, MI, USA
e-mail: aamro1@hfhs.org

L.A. Newman, MD, MPH, FACS, FASCO (✉)
Henry Ford Cancer Institute, Detroit, MI, USA
e-mail: lnewman1@hfhs.org

© Springer International Publishing AG 2018
A.R. Tan (ed.), *Triple-Negative Breast Cancer*,
https://doi.org/10.1007/978-3-319-69980-6_5

55

Therefore standard treatment guidelines feature recommendations for relatively more aggressive management and a lower threshold for adjuvant systemic therapy compared to non-TNBC cases. For example, the National Comprehensive Cancer Network (NCCN) 2017 breast cancer treatment algorithm states that adjuvant chemotherapy should be considered for node-negative TNBC tumors as small as 6–10 mm in size [3]. The association between TNBC and virulent tumor biology also prompts questions regarding optimal locoregional management and whether patients harboring these tumors should receive different surgical options compared to their stage-matched non-TNBC counterparts.

This chapter will summarize the existing literature regarding surgery for TNBC, with a focus on the following issues and questions:

1. Surgical management of the breast:
   (a) Is breast-conserving surgery safe in TNBC patients?
   (b) Is immediate reconstruction safe in TNBC patients undergoing mastectomy?
2. Surgical management of the axilla:
   (a) Is the frequency of nodal involvement higher for TNBC compared to non-TNBC?
   (b) What is the prognostic value of nodal involvement in TNBC?
   (c) Is lymphatic mapping and sentinel lymph node biopsy accurate in patients with TNBC?
3. Neoadjuvant chemotherapy:
   (a) What are the advantages of neoadjuvant chemotherapy in TNBC patients?

5.2 Surgical Management of the Breast in Triple-Negative Breast Cancer

5.2.1 Breast-Conserving Surgery Versus Mastectomy

Several prospective, randomized trials conducted internationally have confirmed that overall survival rates are equivalent for patients undergoing mastectomy surgery compared to those managed by lumpectomy and breast radiation, with survival driven by risk of distant organ metastatic disease, and this surgical approach is endorsed by the NCCN [3, 4]. However, these trials were conducted prior to widespread characterization of invasive breast cancers by biomarker expression, and the virulence of TNBC therefore raises the concern that breast conservation might be associated with a prohibitive excess in risk of local recurrence. Two meta-analyses and several retrospective studies provide important data to address this concern in the context of contemporary breast cancer management accounting for tumor phenotype.

Lowery et al. conducted a systematic review of locoregional recurrence after breast cancer surgery, looking at the impact of biomarker expression [5]. Fifteen studies involving 12,592 patients contributed to this pooled analysis, 7174 of whom

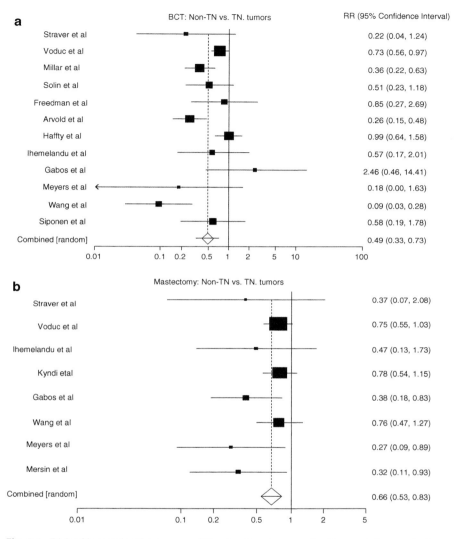

Fig. 5.1 Risk of locoregional recurrence following breast-conserving therapy (**a**) or mastectomy (**b**) in TNBC compared to non-TNBC. From meta-analysis by Lowery et al. [5] (With permission)

underwent breast-conserving surgery and 5418 underwent mastectomy. TNBC was indeed associated with an increased risk of locoregional recurrence, but this correlation was observed regardless of whether mastectomy or breast-conserving surgery was performed. As shown in Fig. 5.1a, b, relative risk of locoregional recurrence for non-TNBC compared to TNBC patients treated with breast conservation was 0.49 (95% confidence interval 0.33–0.73) and 0.66 (95% confidence interval 0.53–0.83) for those undergoing mastectomy. This 2012 meta-analysis notwithstanding, it is worth noting that some recent investigators have reported that TNBC patients do not experience significantly higher rates of locoregional failure compared to non-TNBC patients managed with BCT. Gangi et al. [6] evaluated outcomes among 1851 consecutive BCT patients treated at the Cedars-Sinai Medical Center in California, 234 (12.6%) of whom had TNBC. With median follow-up of 60 months, the 5-year local recurrence-free survival for the TNBC cases was 93% compared to 95%, 96%, and 96% for the luminal A, luminal B, and HER2-overexpressing cases, respectively ($p = 0.13$). Regional recurrence-free survival was 98%, 98%, 96%, and 84% for TNBC, luminal A, luminal B, and HER2-overexpressing cases, respectively ($p < 0.001$).

As summarized in Table 5.1, several studies have furthermore demonstrated that more extensive local surgery in the form of mastectomy for TNBC does not improve likelihood of locoregional control when compared to breast conservation, and some even suggest that lumpectomy with breast radiation achieves better results. Another meta-analysis highlighted the importance of adjuvant radiation therapy in local control for TNBC. O'Rorke et al. [7] reviewed 12 studies involving 5507 TNBC patients (including 6 studies providing locoregional recurrence data in 1795 patients) and reported a pooled hazard ratio for locoregional recurrence of 0.61 (95% confidence interval 0.41–0.90) in the comparison of breast conservation (lumpectomy plus radiation) versus mastectomy (without radiation).

Accordingly, the question of whether mastectomy can overcome the "bad biology" of TNBC and be considered the preferred surgical approach compared to BCT has been reviewed by several experts, including Morrow [8], Pilewskie and King [9], King et al. [10], as well as Chen and Pu [11]. All have concluded that TNBC and non-TNBC patients should be presented the same surgical management options. A case-control study reported by Joyce et al. [12] supports these recommendations. These investigators evaluated 142 TNBC patients matched by age, stage, and Nottingham Prognostic Index to 142 non-TNBC patients. TNBC patients had a survival disadvantage compared to non-TNBC patients (77% of TNBC patients alive at a mean follow-up of 32 months, versus 92% of non-TNBC patients at a mean follow-up of 38 months, $p = 0.0$ Log rank test), but rates of locoregional recurrence were similar in the TNBC patients regardless of whether breast-conserving or mastectomy surgery was performed.

Young, premenopausal breast cancer patients face a disproportionately increased risk of having the TNBC phenotype, and young age at breast cancer diagnosis is also a risk factor for locoregional recurrence. Radosa et al. therefore interrogated the Memorial Sloan Kettering Cancer Center database to determine whether young age at TNBC diagnosis was an indication for mastectomy as a strategy to protect against locoregional recurrence [13]. This study evaluated 289 TNBC patients younger than age 40 years (39% of whom received BCT), compared with 1642 TNBC patients at least age 40 years (58% of whom were managed by BCT). Multivariate analysis revealed that primary tumor size, the presence of lymphovascular invasion, and node positivity were all features associated with an increased risk of locoregional recurrence, but age category and choice of surgery were not.

Table 5.1 Selected studies comparing locoregional recurrence in triple-negative breast cancer patients managed with breast-conserving therapy (lumpectomy and radiation) versus mastectomy (without radiation)

Study, year	Study design	No. TNBC cases	Follow-up	Results
Ihemelandu [40], 2008	Retrospective analysis, African-American patients, Howard University	79	36 months (median)	Multivariate analysis: OR LRR for mastectomy versus BCT 0.81 (95% confidence interval 0.24–2.7; $p = 0.74$) OR LRR TNBC versus non-TNBC 1.0 (95% confidence interval 0.24–4.2; $p = 0.97$)
Parker [41], 2010	Retrospective analysis, two hospitals in Shreveport, LA (USA)	202	52.8 months (mean)	Isolated LR: BCT 0% 10.6% for mastectomy ($p = 0.02$) Isolated RR: BCT—1.6% Mastectomy—1.4% ($p = 0.61$) Multivariate analysis: surgical approach (BCT versus mastectomy) had no effect on DFS or OS
Adkins [42], 2011	Retrospective analysis, MD Anderson Cancer Center (USA)	1325	62 months (median)	5-year LRR-free survival: BCT—76% Mastectomy—71% ($p = 0.032$)
Abdulkarim [43], 2011	Retrospective analysis, Alberta Cancer Registry (Canada)	606	7.2 years (median)	5-year LRR-free survival: BCT—94% Mastectomy—85% ($p < 0.001$) 5-year OS: BCT—87% Mastectomy—82% ($p < 0.001$)
Ly [44], 2012	Retrospective analysis, Jackson Memorial Hospital, FL (USA)	62	40.1 months (median)	7-year cumulative LRR incidence: BCT—19.7% Mastectomy—17.5% ($p = 0.465$) 7-year cumulative DM incidence: BCT—2.63% Mastectomy—22.4% ($p < 0.0001$)
Wang [45], 2013	Meta-analysis	4364	70 months (median)	LRR: BCT—16.9% Mastectomy—21.9% (Relative risk 0.75; 95% confidence interval 0.65–0.87; $p < 0.0001$) DM: BCT—23.6% Mastectomy—34.4% (Relative risk 0.68; 95% confidence interval 0.60–0.76; $p < 0.00001$)

(continued)

Table 5.1 (continued)

Study, year	Study design	No. TNBC cases	Follow-up	Results
Zumsteg [46], 2013	Retrospective analysis; Memorial Sloan Kettering Cancer Center, New York (USA)	646	78.3 months (median)	5-year LRR: BCT—4.2% Mastectomy—5.4% ($p > 0.05$) LRR multivariate analysis: OR LRR mastectomy versus BCT 1.44 (95% confidence interval 0.71–2.92; $p = 0.31$) 5-year cumulative incidence DM: BCT—8.2% Mastectomy—8.1% (HR 0.97; 95% confidence interval 0.54–1.75) OS multivariate analysis: Mastectomy versus BCT HR 1.07 (95% confidence interval 0.64–1.79)
Bhoo-Pathy [16], 2015	Retrospective analysis; five centers in Asia (Malaysia, Singapore, Hong Kong)	1138	T1-2/N0-1 ($n = 775$): 2780 person/year T3-4/N2-3 ($n = 363$): 1166 person/year	5-year relative survival, T1–2/N0–1: BCT—90.8% Mastectomy—94.8% (Adjusted hazard ratio 0.84; 95% confidence interval 0.43–1.65) 5-year relative survival, T3–4/N2–3: BCT—94.1% Mastectomy—58.6% (Adjusted hazard ratio 0.20; 95% confidence interval 0.06–0.60)
Joyce [12], 2016	Case control	142	32 months (mean)	LRR rates described as being similar for BCT and mastectomy cases ($p = 0.449$)
O'Rorke [7], 2016	Meta-analysis	1795	1.9–7.2 years (median)	Hazard ratio LRR BCT versus mastectomy 0.61 (95% confidence interval 0.41–0.90); favoring BCT Hazard ratio OS BCT versus mastectomy 0.57 (95% confidence interval 0.36–0.88); favoring BCT
Chen [47], 2017	Population-based retrospective SEER analysis (USA)	11,514	22 months (median)	Breast cancer-specific survival: BCT better than mastectomy (cumulative survival probability mastectomy versus BCT 0.606; 95% confidence interval 0.502–0.731) Overall survival: BCT better than mastectomy (cumulative survival probability mastectomy versus BCT 0.579; 95% confidence interval 0.488–0.687)

BCT breast-conserving therapy, *No.* number, *OR* odds ratio, *LRR* locoregional recurrence, *LR* local recurrence, *RR* regional recurrence, *SEER* Surveillance, Epidemiology, and End Results

5.2.2 Immediate Reconstruction in Triple-Negative Breast Cancer Patients Undergoing Mastectomy

As noted in the above section and as depicted by the meta-analysis data shown in Fig. 5.1 from Lowery et al., TNBC patients face an increased risk of local as well as distant recurrence, regardless of whether they undergo mastectomy or breast-conserving surgery [5]. The increased risk of chest wall failure following mastectomy then prompts a discussion of whether TNBC should be considered to be an independent indication for postmastectomy radiation (PMRT). Immediate breast reconstruction results can be complicated by the delivery of PMRT [14], with higher risk of implant contracture as well as infection and increased rates of autologous reconstruction fibrosis. While immediate breast reconstruction in PMRT patients has been increasing in frequency, many plastic surgeons continue to prefer delayed reconstruction in patients likely to require PMRT [15]. The question of TNBC as an indication for PMRT therefore remains clinically relevant.

Bhoo-Pathy et al. [16] conducted a historical cohort study involving more than 1000 TNBC patients treated at five centers in Asia and found that PMRT, which was delivered to cases with at least four metastatic lymph nodes or T3/T4 disease, improved outcomes for patients younger than 40 years, but specific data regarding locoregional recurrence were not reported. A subsequent 2016 meta-analysis by O'Rorke et al. [7] confirmed the benefit of PMRT for TNBC cases with regard to locoregional disease control, and provided additional information regarding survival endpoints. Pooled analysis of seven studies revealed that treated cases had a statistically significant improvement in risk of locoregional recurrence compared to patients undergoing mastectomy without radiation (hazard ratio 0.62, 95% confidence interval 0.44–0.88). Six studies contributed data on overall survival (including the Bhoo-Pathy study), revealing no impact of PMRT on distant metastatic risk and longevity. Comparing PMRT to mastectomy without radiation, the hazard ratio for distant metastasis across four studies was 1.40 (95% confidence interval 0.63–3.10); and the hazard ratio for overall survival across six studies was 1.12 (95% confidence interval 0.75–1.69).

The preponderance of the data thus far supports the effectiveness of PMRT in reducing risk of locoregional recurrence among TNBC mastectomy patients that have other indications for considering adjuvant radiation (i.e., locally advanced disease and/or extensive nodal involvement); however, it does not appear to be associated with a survival advantage. Accordingly, neither the St. Gallen International Expert Consensus [17], the European Society of Medical Oncology [18], nor the American Society of Clinical Oncology [19] cites TNBC as an independent indication for PMRT. TNBC patients that are otherwise deemed to be appropriate candidates for immediate reconstruction therefore should not be denied this surgical approach because of concerns regarding PMRT.

5.3   Surgical Management of the Axilla in Triple-Negative Breast Cancer

5.3.1   Frequency of Nodal Metastases for Triple-Negative Breast Cancer Versus Non-Triple-Negative Breast Cancer

The published literature has yielded inconsistent results with regard to TNBC being an independent risk factor for nodal involvement. A 2007 study by Dent et al. [20] raised concerns that risk of regional metastatic extension by TNBC is elevated in comparison to non-TNBC and that this risk is independent of primary tumor size. These investigators reported on frequency of lymph node metastases in 180 TNBC cases stratified by primary tumor size and found rates of 55.6%, 55.6%, 48.9%, and 92.3% in patients with T1b, T1c, T2, and T3 tumors, respectively. In contrast, a recent analysis of more than 38,000 cases from the National Cancer Database found that TNBC tumors had similar frequency of nodal involvement compared to non-TNBC tumors (32.0% versus 31.7%; $p = 0.218$) [21]. Furthermore, on multivariate analysis adjusting for the relatively larger sizes and higher grade of the TNBC cases, a lower risk of node positivity was found (odds ratio 0.59; 95% confidence interval 0.57–0.60). Table 5.2 summarizes studies that have reported on frequency of lymph node involvement for TNBC versus non-TNBC cases.

5.3.2   Prognostic Value of Nodal Metastases in Triple-Negative Breast Cancer

Node-negative TNBC is associated with a relatively worse prognosis compared to node-negative non-TNBC, consistent with the known biologically aggressive nature of these tumors and thereby justifying the lower tumor size threshold for recommending adjuvant chemotherapy even in the absence of regional disease. Metzger-Filho et al. [22] provided data in support of these concepts in their report of nearly 2000 node-negative patients from the International Breast Cancer Study Group trials, including 310 TNBC cases. With a median follow-up of 12.5 years, the 10-year overall survival rates for the luminal A, luminal B, HER2-overexpressing, and TNBC cases were 89%, 83%, 77%, and 75%, respectively.

Despite the inconsistent reported data regarding whether TNBC is more or less likely to be associated with nodal metastases compared to non-TNBC, two large studies have confirmed the prognostic value of whichever nodal status is pathologically documented in these cases. Hernandez-Aya et al. [23] reported on outcomes in 1711 TNBC patients from the University of Texas MD Anderson Cancer Center, with median follow-up of 53 months. Five-year overall survival rates 80%, 65%, 48%, and 44% for patients with N0, N1, N2, and N3 disease, respectively ($p < 0.0001$). Similarly, Wang et al. [24] evaluated survival data from the population-based Surveillance, Epidemiology, and End Results Program. These investigators found the most favorable survival outcomes for the TNBC node-negative patients

Table 5.2 Studies reporting frequency of nodal metastases in triple-negative breast cancer versus non-triple-negative breast cancer

Study, year	No. TNBC cases	Frequency TNBC cases with nodal metastases (%)	No. non-TNBC cases	Frequency non-TNBC cases with nodal metastases	p-Value
Dent [20], 2007	180	54.4	1421	45.6%	0.02
Billar [48], 2010	123	21	ER-positive: 728	ER-positive: 32%	0.025
			HER2-positive: 210	HER2-positive: 37%	
Jones [49], 2013	110	26.8	ER-/PR-positive/ HER2-negative: 220	ER-/PR-positive/ HER2-negative: 22.9%	0.694
			ER-/PR-/HER2-positive: 73	ER-/PR-/HER2-positive: 26.8%	
			ER-/PR-negative/ HER2-positive: 50	ER-/PR-negative/ HER2-positive: 30%	
Howland [50], 2013	65	43.1	ER- and/or PR-positive; HER2-negative; Ki67-low: 95	ER- and/or PR-positive; HER2-negative; Ki67-low: 38.9%	0.0104
			ER- and/or PR-positive; HER2-negative; Ki67-elevated: 120	ER- and/or PR-positive; HER2-negative; Ki67-elevated: 52.5%	
			ER- and/or PR-positive; HER2-positive: 69	ER- and/or PR-positive; HER2-positive: 65.2%	
			ER-/PR-negative; HER2-positive: 26	ER-/PR-negative; HER2-positive: 57.7%	
Plasiliova [21], 2016	33,620	32.0	ER- and/or PR-positive; HER2-negative: 189,125	ER- and/or PR-positive; HER2-negative: 30.3%	0.218
			ER- and/or PR-positive; HER2-positive: 25,694	ER- and/or PR-positive; HER2-positive: 38.2%	
			ER-/PR-negative; HER2-positive: 11,251	ER-/PR-negative; HER2-positive: 40.0%	
Gangi [6], 2016	234	30.5	ER- and/or PR-positive; HER2-negative: 1235	ER- and/or PR-positive; HER2-negative: 24.3%	0.04
			ER- and/or PR-positive; HER2-positive: 194	ER- and/or PR-positive; HER2-positive: 30.4%	
			ER-/PR-negative; HER2-positive: 60	ER-/PR-negative; HER2-positive: 35%	

ER estrogen receptor, PR progesterone receptor, HER2 human epidermal growth factor receptor type 2 and the worst outcomes for patients with at least ten metastatic nodes (N3 disease). Interestingly however, primary tumor size dampened the association between volume of nodal metastases and outcomes in both studies.

5.3.3 Accuracy of Lymphatic Mapping and Sentinel Lymph Node Biopsy in Triple-Negative Breast Cancer

Many of the early studies that evaluated accuracy of lymphatic mapping and sentinel lymph node biopsy by performing a concomitant completion axillary lymph node dissection were conducted prior to the era of routine documentation of HER2 status. It is therefore difficult to definitively assess the false-negative rate of sentinel lymph node biopsy for TNBC cases. Similarly, the American College of Surgeons Z0011 trial [25], which proved the safety of omitting completion axillary lymph node dissection in BCT patients with one or two metastatic sentinel nodes, was based upon a cohort of mostly non-TNBC participants (approximately 83% estrogen receptor-positive and HER2 status not routinely reported for study participants). As described below however, long-term follow-up studies demonstrate low rates of axillary/regional failure among TNBC patients that previously underwent resection of negative sentinel lymph nodes or had limited sentinel node metastatic disease.

Van Roozendaal et al. reported risk of regional recurrence for a Dutch cohort of 2486 TNBC patients diagnosed 2005–2008, and all whom were initially staged via sentinel lymph node biopsy [26]. During 5 years of follow-up, regional recurrences occurred in a total of 75 patients, with approximately 2% occurring among patients that had a negative sentinel lymph node biopsy at time of initial diagnosis.

Mamtani et al. evaluated the safety of extrapolating results from the Z0011 trial to TNBC patients in their report of 701 consecutive BCT patients found to have metastatic sentinel lymph nodes [27]. These cases were categorized as either high risk (including 31 TNBC patients) or average risk. With a median follow-up of 34 months for the high-risk group, no isolated axillary recurrences were detected, despite the fact that completion axillary lymph node dissection was omitted in 85% of cases.

5.4   Neoadjuvant Chemotherapy

As noted previously, the primary tumor size threshold for recommending chemotherapy is lower for the TNBC phenotype compared to hormone receptor-positive disease. Patients with tumors at least 6 mm in size will be candidates for chemotherapy regardless of nodal status [3], and these patients can therefore consider the option of receiving chemotherapy prior to undergoing surgery for their breast cancer. As reviewed by Newman [28], several issues should be addressed before committing the patient to the primary chemotherapy sequence:

(a) To avoid the risk of overtreatment in patients that are clinically node negative, the clinician must be very confident that the size of the invasive tumor component is clearly in the range where chemotherapy will be beneficial. This can be best ascertained by breast imaging consistent with a solid mass larger than 10 mm. Patients whose triple-negative phenotype is detected by core needle biopsy of microcalcifications (in the absence of a solid mass lesion) might actually have microinvasive disease within a span of ductal carcinoma in situ, in which case chemotherapy will not be indicated.

(b) A radiopaque clip should be left at the site of the biopsied tumor mass. Patients that experience a complete clinical response from neoadjuvant chemotherapy still require surgery to the breast, and the clip will serve as a marker for an image-guided lumpectomy in cases where breast conservation is pursued.

(c) Patients that have multiple masses should undergo biopsy of each distinct lesion, with a clip left at each site. Any tumor found to have hormone receptor positivity or HER2 overexpression will serve as an indication for endocrine therapy and targeted anti-HER2 therapy in addition to a generic chemotherapy regimen. Furthermore, the furthest distance between any two tumors will become the rate-limiting factor in deciding on ultimate lumpectomy eligibility. Patients with tumors spaced so far apart that they cannot be resected within a single cosmetically acceptable lumpectomy specimen should be informed that mastectomy is likely to be necessary. The aesthetic acceptability however, must be defined by the patient.

Several factors might strengthen the case in favor of neoadjuvant chemotherapy among TNBC patients presenting with disease that is clearly resectable from a technical perspective: (1) neoadjuvant chemotherapy can reduce the primary tumor size, making the patient a candidate for a smaller-volume lumpectomy; (2) neoadjuvant chemotherapy may sterilize axillary metastases, improving the likelihood that the patient can avoid the morbidity of an axillary lymph node dissection; and (3) neoadjuvant chemotherapy provides the patient with a longer window of time prior to undergoing surgery, thereby giving her an extended timeframe to consider her surgical preferences and potentially complete any necessary genetic counseling and genetic testing. This latter benefit is particularly relevant for TNBC patients, who have an increased risk of harboring a *BRCA* mutation, and genetic counseling is therefore recommended for any TNBC patient ≤60 years of age, regardless of family history [2].

The TNBC phenotype is quite chemosensitive, and these tumors are more likely to achieve a complete pathologic response (pCR) compared to non-TNBC. In a pooled analysis of 12 trials involving nearly 12,000 patients reported by Cortazar et al. [29], neoadjuvant chemotherapy resulted in a pCR for 33.6% of TNBC patients but only 16.2% and 7.5% of hormone receptor-positive/HER2-negative high-grade and non-high-grade cancers, respectively. The seemingly incongruous patterns of TNBC having a higher metastatic risk while also exhibiting higher pCR rates after neoadjuvant chemotherapy (which predicts for improved survival) has been termed the "triple-negative paradox" [30]. Indeed, TNBC and non-TNBC patients achieving a pCR from neoadjuvant chemotherapy have similarly high survival rates, but among the neoadjuvantly treated patients that residual disease, the TNBC cases have a disproportionately poor outcome [31].

For patients presenting with clinically node-negative disease that are triaged to neoadjuvant chemotherapy (including TNBC), NCCN guidelines endorse lymphatic mapping and sentinel lymph node biopsy after treatment, performed concomitantly with the planned breast surgery. The post-neoadjuvant chemotherapy sentinel node-negative patients need not undergo completion axillary lymph node dissection. NCCN guidelines also support opportunities to avoid the axillary lymph node dissection among patients presenting with pathologically confirmed axillary metastases, if a targeted/selective axillary dissection confirms nodal downstaging by the chemotherapy. The targeted axillary dissection is an "enhanced" lymphatic mapping and sentinel lymph node biopsy procedure. It can be performed in neoadjuvant chemotherapy patients whose initial node positivity was confirmed by core needle biopsy, with a clip left in the metastatic lymph node. When the patient undergoes breast and axillary surgery following delivery of the neoadjuvant chemotherapy, dual-agent (blue dye as well as radioactive tracer) mapping is performed, and at least two or three mapped sentinel node(s) must be resected, with inclusion of the originally biopsied/clipped node confirmed by axillary specimen mammography. Regardless of whether the clipped node is identified by wire localization, seed localization, or palpation, radiographic confirmation that the originally biopsied node has been resected is mandatory. While past clinical trials [32, 33] and retrospective studies [34–36] have revealed unacceptably high sentinel node false-negative rates when routine lymphatic mapping is performed after neoadjuvant chemotherapy, the targeted dissection reduces these rates to less than 7% [37, 38]. Completion axillary lymph node dissection and regional radiation are the current standard of care management for patients found to have residual sentinel node metastases following neoadjuvant chemotherapy, but the Alliance A11202 trial [39] is exploring alternatives by randomizing these patients to either axillary dissection plus regional radiation or to regional radiation alone.

5.5   Summary

In conclusion, the medical literature thus far supports the following answers to the previously proposed questions:

1. Surgical management of the breast:
   (a) Is breast-conserving surgery safe in TNBC patients?
       Yes. TNBC patients have an increased risk of distant metastatic failure that is not mitigated by mastectomy surgery and local control rates are acceptable following BCT (lumpectomy and radiation).
   (b) Is immediate reconstruction safe in TNBC patients undergoing mastectomy?
       Yes. Despite the data from some studies indicating higher rates of chest wall failure in TNBC patients undergoing mastectomy, TNBC is not an independent risk factor for postmastectomy radiation, and decisions regarding eligibility for immediate reconstruction should not be based upon phenotype alone.
2. Surgical management of the axilla:
   (a) Is the frequency of nodal involvement higher for TNBC compared to non-TNBC?

The reported literature yields inconsistent results with regard to whether TNBC is an independent risk factor for axillary metastatic disease.

(b) What is the prognostic value of nodal involvement in TNBC?

Nodal status retains its prognostic value among TNBC patients, and these patients should therefore continue to undergo axillary staging.

(c) Is lymphatic mapping and sentinel lymph node biopsy accurate in patients with TNBC?

Yes. While data regarding quantified false-negative rates for sentinel lymph node biopsy in TNBC cases are limited, long-term follow-up studies reveal low rates of axillary recurrence among TNBC patients managed by resection of a negative sentinel lymph node biopsy alone at time of initial diagnosis. TNBC patients managed by BCT (lumpectomy followed by whole-breast radiation) and found to have metastatic disease in one or two sentinel lymph nodes can be managed similar to non-TNBC patients and can safely avoid completion axillary lymph node dissection.

3. What are the advantages of neoadjuvant chemotherapy in TNBC patients?

TNBC patients tend to respond briskly to neoadjuvant chemotherapy. This treatment sequence can improve lumpectomy eligibility as well as downstage the axilla, thereby making axillary lymph node dissection less likely. The neoadjuvant chemotherapy delivery interval also provides the patient with a window of time for consideration of breast surgical preferences and completion of genetic counseling and testing.

References

1. Hudis CA, Gianni L. Triple-negative breast cancer: an unmet medical need. Oncologist. 2011;16(Suppl 1):1–11.
2. Newman LA, Reis-Filho JS, Morrow M, Carey LA, King TA. The 2014 Society of Surgical Oncology Susan G. Komen for the Cure Symposium: triple-negative breast cancer. Ann Surg Oncol. 2015;22(3):874–82.
3. National Comprehensive Cancer Network Version 1.2017, 03/10/17 at https://www.nccn.org/professionals/physician_gls/pdf/breast.pdf. Last accessed 29 March 2017.
4. Newman LA. Decision making in the surgical management of invasive breast cancer-part 1: lumpectomy, mastectomy, and contralateral prophylactic mastectomy. Oncology. 2017;31(5):359–68.
5. Lowery AJ, Kell MR, Glynn RW, Kerin MJ, Sweeney KJ. Locoregional recurrence after breast cancer surgery: a systematic review by receptor phenotype. Breast Cancer Res Treat. 2012;133(3):831–41.
6. Gangi A, Chung A, Mirocha J, Liou DZ, Leong T, Giuliano AE. Breast-conserving therapy for triple-negative breast cancer. JAMA Surg. 2014;149(3):252–8.
7. O'Rorke MA, Murray LJ, Brand JS, Bhoo-Pathy N. The value of adjuvant radiotherapy on survival and recurrence in triple-negative breast cancer: a systematic review and meta-analysis of 5507 patients. Cancer Treat Rev. 2016;47:12–21.
8. Morrow M. Personalizing extent of breast cancer surgery according to molecular subtypes. Breast. 2013;22(Suppl 2):S106–9.
9. Pilewskie M, King TA. Age and molecular subtypes: impact on surgical decisions. J Surg Oncol. 2014;110(1):8–14.
10. King TA, Pilewskie M, Morrow M. Optimal surgical management for high-risk populations. Breast. 2015;24(Suppl 2):S91–5.

11. Chen F, Pu F. Role of postmastectomy radiotherapy in early-stage (T1-2N0-1M0) triple-negative breast cancer: a systematic review. Onco Targets Ther. 2017;10:2009–16.
12. Joyce DP, Murphy D, Lowery AJ, et al. Prospective comparison of outcome after treatment for triple-negative and non-triple-negative breast cancer. Surgeon. 2017;15:272–7.
13. Radosa JC, Eaton A, Stempel M, et al. Evaluation of local and distant recurrence patterns in patients with triple-negative breast cancer according to age. Ann Surg Oncol. 2017;24:698–704.
14. Kronowitz SJ, Robb GL. Radiation therapy and breast reconstruction: a critical review of the literature. Plast Reconstr Surg. 2009;124(2):395–408.
15. Clemens MW, Kronowitz SJ. Current perspectives on radiation therapy in autologous and prosthetic breast reconstruction. Gland Surg. 2015;4(3):222–31.
16. Bhoo-Pathy N, Verkooijen HM, Wong FY, et al. Prognostic role of adjuvant radiotherapy in triple-negative breast cancer: a historical cohort study. Int J Cancer. 2015;137:2504–12.
17. Morigi C. Highlights from the 15th St Gallen International Breast Cancer Conference 15-18 March, 2017, Vienna: tailored treatments for patients with early breast cancer. Ecancermedicalscience. 2017;11:732.
18. Senkus E, Kyriakides S, Penault-Llorca F, et al. Primary breast cancer: ESMO Clinical Practice Guidelines for diagnosis, treatment and follow-up. Ann Oncol. 2013;24(Suppl 6):vi7–23.
19. Recht A, Comen EA, Fine RE, et al. Postmastectomy radiotherapy: an American Society of Clinical Oncology, American Society for Radiation Oncology, and Society of Surgical Oncology Focused Guideline Update. J Clin Oncol. 2016;34(36):4431–42.
20. Dent R, Trudeau M, Pritchard KI, et al. Triple-negative breast cancer: clinical features and patterns of recurrence. Clin Cancer Res. 2007;13(15 Pt 1):4429–34.
21. Plasilova ML, Hayse B, Killelea BK, Horowitz NR, Chagpar AB, Lannin DR. Features of triple-negative breast cancer: analysis of 38,813 cases from the national cancer database. Medicine. 2016;95(35):e4614.
22. Metzger-Filho O, Sun Z, Viale G, et al. Patterns of Recurrence and outcome according to breast cancer subtypes in lymph node-negative disease: results from international breast cancer study group trials VIII and IX. J Clin Oncol. 2013;31(25):3083–90.
23. Hernandez-Aya LF, Chavez-Macgregor M, Lei X, et al. Nodal status and clinical outcomes in a large cohort of patients with triple-negative breast cancer. J Clin Oncol. 2011;29:2628–34.
24. Wang XX, Jiang YZ, Li JJ, Song CG, Shao ZM. Effect of nodal status on clinical outcomes of triple-negative breast cancer: a population-based study using the SEER 18 database. Oncotarget. 2016;7:46636–45.
25. Giuliano AE, Ballman K, McCall L, et al. Locoregional recurrence after sentinel lymph node dissection with or without axillary dissection in patients with sentinel lymph node metastases: long-term follow-up from the American College of Surgeons Oncology Group (Alliance) ACOSOG Z0011 Randomized Trial. Ann Surg. 2016;264(3):413–20.
26. van Roozendaal LM, Smit LH, Duijsens GH, et al. Risk of regional recurrence in triple-negative breast cancer patients: a Dutch cohort study. Breast Cancer Res Treat. 2016;156(3):465–72.
27. Mamtani A, Patil S, Van Zee KJ, et al. Age and receptor status do not indicate the need for axillary dissection in patients with sentinel lymph node metastases. Ann Surg Oncol. 2016;23(11):3481–6.
28. Newman LA. Decision making in the surgical management of invasive breast cancer-part 2: expanded applications for breast-conserving surgery. Oncology. 2017;31(5):415–20.
29. Cortazar P, Zhang L, Untch M, et al. Pathological complete response and long-term clinical benefit in breast cancer: the CTNeoBC pooled analysis. Lancet. 2014;384:164–72.
30. Carey LA, Dees EC, Sawyer L, et al. The triple negative paradox: primary tumor chemosensitivity of breast cancer subtypes. Clin Cancer Res. 2007;13(8):2329–34.
31. Liedtke C, Mazouni C, Hess KR, et al. Response to neoadjuvant therapy and long-term survival in patients with triple-negative breast cancer. J Clin Oncol. 2008;26(8):1275–81.
32. Boughey JC, Suman VJ, Mittendorf EA, et al. Sentinel lymph node surgery after neoadjuvant chemotherapy in patients with node-positive breast cancer: the ACOSOG Z1071 (Alliance) clinical trial. JAMA. 2013;310(14):1455–61.

33. Kuehn T, Bauerfeind I, Fehm T, et al. Sentinel-lymph-node biopsy in patients with breast cancer before and after neoadjuvant chemotherapy (SENTINA): a prospective, multicentre cohort study. Lancet Oncol. 2013;14(7):609–18.
34. van Deurzen CH, Vriens BE, Tjan-Heijnen VC, et al. Accuracy of sentinel node biopsy after neoadjuvant chemotherapy in breast cancer patients: a systematic review. Eur J Cancer. 2009;45(18):3124–30.
35. Kelly AM, Dwamena B, Cronin P, Carlos RC. Breast cancer sentinel node identification and classification after neoadjuvant chemotherapy-systematic review and meta analysis. Acad Radiol. 2009;16(5):551–63.
36. Xing Y, Foy M, Cox DD, Kuerer HM, Hunt KK, Cormier JN. Meta-analysis of sentinel lymph node biopsy after preoperative chemotherapy in patients with breast cancer. Br J Surg. 2006;93(5):539–46.
37. Caudle AS, Yang WT, Krishnamurthy S, et al. Improved axillary evaluation following neoadjuvant therapy for patients with node-positive breast cancer using selective evaluation of clipped nodes: implementation of targeted axillary dissection. J Clin Oncol. 2016;34(10):1072–8.
38. Boughey JC, Ballman KV, Le-Petross HT, et al. Identification and resection of clipped node decreases the false-negative rate of sentinel lymph node surgery in patients presenting with node-positive breast cancer (T0-T4, N1-N2) who receive neoadjuvant chemotherapy: results from ACOSOG Z1071 (Alliance). Ann Surg. 2016;263(4):802–7.
39. Alliance 11202-comparison of axillary lymph node dissection with axillary radiation for patients with node-positive breast cancer treated with chemotherapy. https://clinicaltrials.gov/ct2/show/NCT01901094. Last accessed 30 May 2017.
40. Ihemelandu CU, Naab TJ, Mezghebe HM, et al. Basal cell-like (triple-negative) breast cancer, a predictor of distant metastasis in African American women. Am J Surg. 2008;195(2):153–8.
41. Parker CC, Ampil F, Burton G, Li BD, Chu QD. Is breast conservation therapy a viable option for patients with triple-receptor negative breast cancer? Surgery. 2010;148(2):386–91.
42. Adkins FC, Gonzalez-Angulo AM, Lei X, et al. Triple-negative breast cancer is not a contraindication for breast conservation. Ann Surg Oncol. 2011;18(11):3164–73.
43. Abdulkarim BS, Cuartero J, Hanson J, Deschenes J, Lesniak D, Sabri S. Increased risk of locoregional recurrence for women with T1-2N0 triple-negative breast cancer treated with modified radical mastectomy without adjuvant radiation therapy compared with breast-conserving therapy. J Clin Oncol. 2011;29(21):2852–8.
44. Ly B, Kwon D, Reis I, et al. Comparison of clinical outcomes in early stage triple negative breast cancer patients treated with mastectomy versus breast conserving therapy. Int J Radiat Oncol Biol Phys. 2012;84(3S):S259–60.
45. Wang J, Xie X, Wang X, et al. Locoregional and distant recurrences after breast conserving therapy in patients with triple-negative breast cancer: a meta-analysis. Surg Oncol. 2013;22(4):247–55.
46. Zumsteg ZS, Morrow M, Arnold B, et al. Breast-conserving therapy achieves locoregional outcomes comparable to mastectomy in women with T1-2N0 triple-negative breast cancer. Ann Surg Oncol. 2013;20(11):3469–76.
47. Chen QX, Wang XX, Lin PY, et al. The different outcomes between breast-conserving surgery and mastectomy in triple-negative breast cancer: a population-based study from the SEER 18 database. Oncotarget. 2017;8(3):4773–80.
48. Billar JA, Dueck AC, Stucky CC, et al. Triple-negative breast cancers: unique clinical presentations and outcomes. Ann Surg Oncol. 2010;17(Suppl 3):384–90.
49. Jones T, Neboori H, Wu H, et al. Are breast cancer subtypes prognostic for nodal involvement and associated with clinicopathologic features at presentation in early-stage breast cancer? Ann Surg Oncol. 2013;20(9):2866–72.
50. Howland NK, Driver TD, Sedrak MP, et al. Lymph node involvement in immunohistochemistry-based molecular classifications of breast cancer. J Surg Res. 2013;185(2):697–703.

Radiation Therapy for Triple-Negative Breast Cancer

6

Suzanne B. Evans and Bruce G. Haffty

Clinical Pearls
- Radiation therapy after lumpectomy is effective at decreasing the risk of locoregional recurrence in triple-negative breast cancer patients.
- Partial breast radiation for triple-negative tumors is not well supported by the current data.
- At present, the indications for postmastectomy radiation therapy are not significantly altered in the setting of triple-negative breast cancer.

6.1 Overview of Radiation Therapy in the Management of Triple-Negative Breast Cancer

The role of radiation therapy in the management of breast cancer is well-established, with numerous randomized trials establishing radiation as a modality which decreases locoregional relapse and increases overall survival, both in the setting of mastectomy and breast conservation therapy [1–3]. Although TNBC constitutes 15–20% of breast cancer presently [4], human epidermal growth factor receptor type 2 (HER2) testing became widely used only in the early twenty-first century, and so the prevalence of this entity in the composition of the early radiotherapeutic trials is unclear. TNBC has associations with several demographic and social factors, which have changed over time, opening the possibility that its prevalence

S.B. Evans, MD, MPH (✉)
Department of Therapeutic Radiology, Yale University School of Medicine,
New Haven, CT, USA
e-mail: suzanne.evans@yale.edu

B.G. Haffty, MD, FASTRO
Department of Radiation Oncology, Rutgers Cancer Institute of New Jersey
and Rutgers Robert Wood Johnson Medical School, New Brunswick, NJ, USA
e-mail: hafftybg@cinj.rutgers.edu

© Springer International Publishing AG 2018
A.R. Tan (ed.), *Triple-Negative Breast Cancer*,
https://doi.org/10.1007/978-3-319-69980-6_6

in prior years may have been different from today. TNBC has associations with *BRCA1* status [5], as well as obesity, age [6], and African American race [7–9]. Traditionally protective factors for breast cancer, like early parity and multiparity, actually may increase the risk for TNBC [10]. Because of these uncertainties, some investigators have questioned the applicability of these earlier studies in radiation to TNBC.

In addition to the potential underrepresentation of TNBC in early radiotherapeutic trials, TNBC has a distinct natural history. TNBC has been shown to have higher rates of local failure when compared to irradiated patients with luminal-type cancers or HER2-enriched cancers that have received HER2-directed therapy. This local recurrence risk may be accentuated in the presence of obesity [11]. Additionally, TNBC patterns of distant recurrence differ, with less bony metastases and more central nervous system [12] and pulmonary metastases, particularly early in the course of disease. Overall recurrence risk peaks within the first 3 years and is quite uncommon after 5 years [13]. Despite these general observations, it has been postulated that TNBC may be a heterogeneous population, with variants such as basaloid with expression of basal keratins, BRCA1 dysfunction with mutations or gene silencing, androgen receptor expression, epidermal growth factor receptor (EGFR) overexpression, and other as yet characterized variants [14]. For the purposes of this discussion, these subtleties will not be explored.

Despite the difference between TNBC and other subtypes, radiation remains a useful tool in the management of TNBC, both in the adjuvant and palliative settings. When considering the importance of locoregional therapy in TNBC, it is helpful to consider the inverted U-shaped curve of the benefit of local radiotherapy by Puglia et al. [15] (Fig. 6.1). Given the nascent state of systemic therapy for TNBC and the persistent problem of inadequate systemic therapy resulting in death from distant disease, local therapy may not predominate as the

Fig. 6.1 A hypothetical U-shaped curve as suggested by Punglia et al. [15]. In this schema, the effect of local therapy is maximized in the era of effective systemic therapy, where distant metastatic failure rates are low, allowing for a profound effect of local therapy on overall survival. At the far end of the curve, with maximally effective systemic therapy, local therapy would have less of a role in management (used with permission)

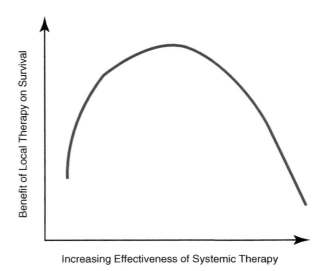

disease modifying element. It may be that the role of radiation for triple-negative breast cancer expands as systemic therapy improves, until the point of maximally effective systemic therapy, which has yet to be reached even for luminal A cancers.

6.2 Triple-Negative Breast Cancer and Management of the Breast

Following lumpectomy with radiation, women with TNBC have been shown to have inferior outcomes when compared to women with luminal cancers. Early studies examining local recurrence and subtype following BCT were in an era before there was effective HER2-directed therapy, which may have been responsible for the potentially misleading lack of difference in local recurrence in TNBC when compared to other subtypes [16]. Local recurrence in the setting of BCT for women with TNBC is reported at 7.1–15.3% versus 0.8–4.3% for luminal cancers [17, 18]. Given the aggressive nature of TNBC and predilection for recurrence [19], many have wondered whether more aggressive surgery is warranted in these cases. In answer to this, an analysis of women with T1 and T2 N0 TNBC who received mastectomy or lumpectomy (per patient choice) showed that those with mastectomy had an inferior local control outcome to breast conservation therapy [20]. Additionally, a single institution analysis examined women treated with BCT, mastectomy, or mastectomy with radiation in TNBC [21]. In this analysis, mastectomy with radiation had significantly lower LRR when compared with the mastectomy alone group or the breast conservation therapy group. Survival was significantly worse in those women with TNBC who received mastectomy alone. Therefore, it seems that BCT is appropriate in women with TNBC.

6.3 Triple-Negative Breast Cancer and Surgical Excision: Considerations of Margins

The appropriate surgical margin for women undergoing lumpectomy in the setting of whole breast radiation therapy has also been examined. The joint guidelines which proposed the standard that in invasive disease, no tumor on ink was sufficient margin, also addressed the question of whether more extensive tumor clearance is warranted in women with TNBC [22]. A retrospective study of approximately 500 patients specifically addressed this question, with margins >2 mm having similar rates of local recurrence [23]. It should be noted that this population was predominantly T1c tumors and chemotherapy use also predominated (76–86%) and that the reported LR rates of 4.7% for margins <2 mm and 3.7% for margins >2 mm, respectively, are lower than rates reported in other series. Reviewing the evidence, it was concluded that greater excision margins did not ameliorate the higher observed local failure rate.

6.4   Timing of Radiotherapy in Triple-Negative Breast Cancer

With regard to the administration of radiation, there is data to suggest that the surgery to radiotherapy interval should be minimized in women not receiving chemotherapy [24–26]. Radiobiologically, it would seem that this surgery to radiation therapy delay results in tumor cell repopulation between surgery and RT, resulting in inferior local control. Given the rapid rate of growth of TNBC, it is logical to assume that this would hold particularly true for women with this disease. However, whether or not the hazard ratio for local recurrence in the presence of delay might differ among TNBC and luminal cancers is unknown. The majority of patients with TNBC receive chemotherapy, and RT should be administered within 2–6 weeks after chemotherapy. For the minority of patients who do not receive chemotherapy, administration of RT within 3–6 weeks of surgery is prudent. The aforementioned time frames are estimated, and each clinic may find that their practice differs from these parameters. The key takeaway is that there remains insufficient data to guide clinicians as to how much of a delay is too long in the specific setting of TNBC, and every effort should be made to avoid delayed administration of RT.

6.5   The Use of the Tumor Bed Boost in Triple-Negative Breast Cancer

Standard practice among women with invasive breast cancer is inclusive of boost to the surgical bed. Given the baseline higher rate of local recurrence in TNBC, boost becomes particularly important for this cohort of women in terms of maximal risk reduction. Multiple trials have shown a benefit in reduction of local recurrence with this strategy. The EORTC boost versus no boost trial [27, 28] showed a hazard reduction of 0.65 for recurrence with the use of boost. Long-term follow-up of this trial [27], looking at prognostic factors, used hormone-receptor-negative tumors with high grade as a surrogate for TNBC, as HER2 status was not available. This trial specifically examined the HR for boost in this population on 15-year risk of IBTR and found that boost conferred a HR of 0.23 ($P = 0.01$). It should be noted that this population had low rates of systemic therapy usage, and this should be considered when calculating the possible benefit of boost in the modern era for these women. For women with TNBC, the ability to localize the tumor bed for boost is arguably more important than for women with luminal A disease, given the higher absolute benefit to this strategy. Placement of surgical clips at the lumpectomy bed is advisable to facilitate tumor bed localization, particularly for those with concurrent oncoplastic reduction or a closed surgical bed technique.

6.6 Target Volumes in Triple-Negative Breast Cancer

The European Society for Radiotherapy and Oncology (ESTRO) consensus guideline was developed primarily for early-stage disease, and as such, the contouring target volumes developed differed from the Radiation Therapy Oncology Group volume guidelines and tended to be smaller in their volume [29]. An analysis of this data revealed a trend toward increased failure in TNBC patients outside of the ESTRO clinical target volumes. However, this did not reach statistical significance. At present, there is no indication to modify standard treatment fields for triple-negative disease.

6.7 The Use of Hypofractionation in Triple-Negative Breast Cancer

The United Kingdom Start B trial examined the use of 4005 cGy in 15 fractions versus 5000 cGy in 25 fractions [30]. Tamoxifen use was recorded in the trial, but estrogen receptor status was not. Standard practice included tamoxifen for ER-positive patients. Approximately 87% in both arms received tamoxifen, with or without chemotherapy, so it seems that the ER-negative, potentially triple-negative (or HER2-enriched) tumors could not have made up more than 13% of the study population. As such, a criticism of the applicability of hypofractionation to TNBC has been their apparent underrepresentation on these trials. The initial Whelan trial [31] raised concern that an unplanned subset analysis suggested less effectiveness with hypofractionation in grade 3 tumors. However, the grading system used in that trial is now no longer employed, and this was not validated in other trials [32]. In a retrospective classification through analysis of tissue-banked specimens (80.1%) on the Canadian study [33], tumors were classified as luminal A, luminal B, basal-like, or HER2-enriched. With 12-year follow-up, molecular subtype was the only factor predictive of local recurrence. Interestingly, in this analysis, basal-like (TNBC) had the same LR as luminal A tumors at 4.5%. This is hypothesis-generating data, as it seems to suggest that there is no decrement and possibly an improvement in local control with the use of hypofractionated regimens in this population. It is interesting to note that in this subset analysis, luminal B tumors and HER2-positive tumors had LR as one would expect in the pre-HER2-targeted therapy era, and it was only TNBC that was the outlier (7.9% and 16.1%, respectively). However, the small patient numbers of the basal-like cohort ($n = 125$, 12.6%) prevent definitive conclusions. The American Society for Radiation Oncology (ASTRO) consensus guidelines [34] are currently under revision. The 2011 guideline did not reach consensus on the use of hypofractionation in patients receiving chemotherapy, though most of the authors of the guideline acknowledged treating patients who received chemotherapy with hypofractionation. Since more data is now available on the use of chemotherapy with hypofractionation, this issue will likely be revisited in the whole breast fractionation guideline under development.

6.8   Partial Breast Radiation and Triple-Negative Breast Cancer

Women with early-stage TNBC who are interested in minimizing their exposure to RT and maximizing convenience may be tempted to consider partial breast radiation. However, this population has been underrepresented on trials of partial breast radiation. A study examining interstitial brachytherapy found that local recurrence happened in 11.3% of TNBC, compared to 3.5% risk of luminal A cancers [35], although this finding has not been universally reproduced [36]. Additionally, smaller series have shown that TNBC was associated with higher absolute risks of recurrence, consistent with the whole breast radiation experience. The randomized data [37] from interstitial brachytherapy showed overall excellent results; however, TNBC was underrepresented on this trial. Given the association between local recurrence and survival, such decrements as observed with TNBC and APBI are concerning, and the ideal management of women with TNBC would enroll them on clinical trial if APBI is desired.

6.9   Triple-Negative Breast Cancer in Older Women

Age has long been recognized as a powerful prognostic factor in outcomes among women with breast cancer, with younger age typically portending a worse prognosis, despite otherwise bland-appearing pathology. Additionally, nearly one-third of cases occur in women aged over 70 [38]. Given this, the clinical question that often arises is whether older age is protective against adverse pathology, such as triple-negative disease. A retrospective analysis of women aged 70 and older [39] examined this question. In examining distant disease-free survival in women aged 70–74, 75–79, and >80 years of age, molecular subtype (TNBC- and HER2-positive) was found to be significant, rather than advancing age. Additionally, there is data to suggest that lymph node involvement may be more likely in women over 70 [40], with the hypothesis that poorer immune function in older women may be responsible for this phenomenon. Furthermore, recent advances in survival and outcomes have left older women unaffected by this positive turn [41], perhaps because of decreased adjuvant chemotherapy use, even in "fit" older women [42]. Given these observations, the assumption that TNBC in older women will behave indolently is unwarranted. Adjuvant radiation should be administered as indicated, within the context of a comprehensive geriatric assessment.

6.10   Triple-Negative Breast Cancer and Management of the Regional Nodes

With regard to regional nodal management, there have been substantial changes in recent history. Data regarding TNBC does not suggest that these cancers have a greater propensity for regional nodal metastasis [43, 44]. The ACOSOG Z0011 trial [45] and the After Mapping of the Axilla: Radiation or Surgery (AMAROS) trial [46] have led to decreased axillary dissections in patients with clinical node-negative disease. Although these trials had relatively few triple-negative patients enrolled (16% ER- and PR-negative in both arms of Z0011, not reported in AMAROS), consistent with the decreased prevalence of this disease, there was no suggestion that this data did not apply to women with TNBC. Hormone-receptor-positive status was associated with a HR of 0.30 ($P = 0.002$) for locoregional failure but was consistent in both arms, suggestive that this was driven by underlying biology rather than treatment strategy. Therefore, in women with clinically negative nodes and TNBC, findings of one or two positive sentinel nodes do not mandate axillary dissection. Consistent with the trial eligibility, women with T1 and T2 tumors who are clinically node negative but (limited) sentinel node positive may safely avoid axillary dissection, even in the presence of TNBC.

There has been considerable debate among radiation oncologists about the importance of treatment of internal mammary nodes. While an earlier study failed to show a significant survival benefit to irradiation of the internal mammary nodes [47], this trial was underpowered. The MA20 trial [48] and the EORTC trial [49] included radiation to the supraclavicular, internal mammary, and undissected level II and III axillary nodes. While neither trial showed statistically significant improved survival from this strategy, they both reported improved disease-free survival and distant disease-free survival with regional nodal RT. In particular, it should be noted that women with hormone-receptor-negative disease in the MA20 trial did show improved survival. Given this data, a strategy of regional nodal radiation is particularly favored in this population.

6.11   The Role of Pathologic Complete Response in Locoregional Decision Making in Triple-Negative Breast Cancer

Women with TNBC who undergo neoadjuvant chemotherapy have enhanced rates of pathologic complete response, and survival is favorably improved with this [50]. There is data to suggest that in TNBC women treated with neoadjuvant chemotherapy who achieve pathologic complete response, there is a favorable impact on LRR in the setting of BCT [51], approximating that of their non-TNBC peers. While the utility of radiation in women with pathologic complete response in breast conservation is clear, there has been considerable interest in the potential elimination of PMRT in women with N1 disease who undergo neoadjuvant chemotherapy with pathology complete response, based on low rates of local failure observed in 100 women treated on trial without PMRT [52]. Presently the National Surgical Adjuvant Breast and Bowel Project has an ongoing trial investigating this question. In the interim, there is insufficient data to suggest that PMRT can be avoided in these women.

6.12   The Use of Postmastectomy Radiation in Triple-Negative Breast Cancer

The Early Breast Cancer Trialists' Collaborative Group has shown benefit in node-positive women to postmastectomy radiation, even in the setting of a single positive node [3]. In this trial, overall recurrence, locoregional recurrence, and breast cancer mortality were positively impacted by the addition of radiation, even in the presence of systemic therapy. The relative risk for breast cancer mortality was 0.78 in women receiving systemic therapy, 0.80 in women with one to three positive nodes, and 0.87 in women with four or more positive nodes. Note that the benefit in breast cancer mortality was actually more dramatic in women receiving systemic therapy and with a lesser nodal burden, consistent with the Punglia hypothetical curve [15] regarding the relationship between distant metastatic risk/effectiveness of systemic therapy and benefit of local therapy. Some concern may be raised over data [53] which suggests a lower absolute benefit to PMRT in women treated on the Danish postmastectomy trials 82b and 82c. This analysis suggested that women with TNBC, the overall survival benefit was lacking (39% versus 32%), and the absolute reduction in locoregional recurrence was 17%. Although these patients received chemotherapy in the form of cyclophosphamide, methotrexate, and fluorouracil, this dismal overall survival in this predominantly node-positive population indicates that systemic therapy was not optimal, thereby limiting the ability of radiotherapy to impact overall survival. A similar analysis [54] of this data divided women into subgroups: a "good" designation was assigned to women with at least four out of five favorable criteria (<3 positive nodes, tumor size <2 cm, grade 1 malignancy, estrogen or progesterone receptor positive, HER2 negative), a "poor" subgroup defined by at least two out of three unfavorable criteria (>3 positive nodes, tumor size >5 cm, grade 3 malignancy), and an "intermediate" which is the group in between. This division of the population revealed that women with the poorest expectations of local control actually had the least survival benefit to RT (Fig. 6.2). As ER-negative, grade 3 patients (TNBC) would fall into the "poor" category where systemic failure dominates, it is not surprising that local therapy may fail to improve outcomes. A meta-analysis of 12 trials of TNBC compared BCT or PMRT to mastectomy alone [55]. In this analysis, the use of PMRT versus mastectomy alone was associated with a hazard ratio for local recurrence of 0.62, although overall survival benefit was not observed. As modern systemic therapy continues to reduce distant failures, clinicians should take care to avoid therapeutic nihilism and continue to offer PMRT in eligible women with TNBC.

6.13   Is TNBC Alone an Indication for Postmastectomy Radiation Therapy?

Given the higher rates of LRR among this subtype, several investigators have conducted analyses on patients with TNBC not usually considered for PMRT. An analysis of T1-2 N0 patients treated with mastectomy [56] revealed that LRR was acceptably low without RT in women treated with mastectomy alone (1.9%),

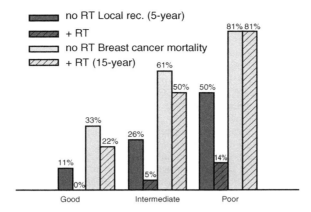

Fig. 6.2 Relationship between overall survival (lighter grey bars), locoregional recurrence (darker grey bars), and prognostic group in the setting of postmastectomy radiation and CMF chemotherapy [54]. Note that in an era of what would today be considered inferior systemic therapy, overall survival benefit to RT was seen predominantly in the better-prognosis patients (used with permission)

although they noted that in women with close or positive margins, LRR was 12.5%. A retrospective analysis from a single institution also examined women with TNBC with T1-2 N0 disease [57] and found that locoregional recurrence-free survival was excellent without radiation (92.9%). An intriguing study [58] examined the role of RT in women with stage I and II TNBC following mastectomy. In this study, 70% were stage I disease, and 5-year overall survival was improved in the radiation arm by nearly 12%. However, this trial is lacking data on RT methods, as well an absence of detail of locoregional recurrence patterns. As such, this trial has had little impact on current practice guidelines.

Conclusions

TNBC poses a management challenge as it has a unique natural history with a propensity for recurrence not observed in other subtypes. At this time, modifying locoregional management decisions based on subtype alone is not supported by the data. These authors advocate for the use of radiation in accordance with the current standard of care, and considerable caution should be used when employing more novel treatment approaches.

References

1. Fisher B, et al. Twenty-year follow-up of a randomized trial comparing total mastectomy, lumpectomy, and lumpectomy plus irradiation for the treatment of invasive breast cancer. N Engl J Med. 2002;347(16):1233–41.
2. Early Breast Cancer Trialists' Collaborative Group. Effect of radiotherapy after breast-conserving surgery on 10-year recurrence and 15-year breast cancer death: meta-analysis of individual patient data for 10 801 women in 17 randomised trials. Lancet. 2011;378(9804):1707–16.

3. McGale P, et al. Effect of radiotherapy after mastectomy and axillary surgery on 10-year recurrence and 20-year breast cancer mortality: meta-analysis of individual patient data for 8135 women in 22 randomised trials. Lancet. 2014;383(9935):2127–35.
4. Zaky SS, et al. The negative effect of triple-negative breast cancer on outcome after breast-conserving therapy. Ann Surg Oncol. 2011;18(10):2858–65.
5. Gonzalez-Angulo AM, et al. Incidence and outcome of BRCA mutations in unselected patients with triple receptor-negative breast cancer. Clin Cancer Res. 2011;17(5):1082–9.
6. Kwan ML, et al. Epidemiology of breast cancer subtypes in two prospective cohort studies of breast cancer survivors. Breast Cancer Res. 2009;11(3):R31.
7. Carey LA, et al. Race, breast cancer subtypes, and survival in the Carolina Breast Cancer Study. JAMA. 2006;295(21):2492–502.
8. Lakhani SR, et al. The pathology of familial breast cancer: predictive value of immunohistochemical markers estrogen receptor, progesterone receptor, HER-2, and p53 in patients with mutations in BRCA1 and BRCA2. J Clin Oncol. 2002;20(9):2310–8.
9. Moran MS, et al. Long-term outcomes and clinicopathologic differences of African-American versus white patients treated with breast conservation therapy for early-stage breast cancer. Cancer. 2008;113(9):2565–74.
10. Ray M, Polite BN. Triple-negative breast cancers: a view from 10,000 feet. Cancer J. 2010;16(1):17–22.
11. Widschwendter P, et al. The influence of obesity on survival in early, high-risk breast cancer: results from the randomized SUCCESS A trial. Breast Cancer Res. 2015;17:129.
12. Heitz F, et al. Triple-negative and HER2-overexpressing breast cancers exhibit an elevated risk and an earlier occurrence of cerebral metastases. Eur J Cancer. 2009;45(16):2792–8.
13. Dent R, et al. Triple-negative breast cancer: clinical features and patterns of recurrence. Clin Cancer Res. 2007;13(15 Pt 1):4429–34.
14. Elias AD. Triple-negative breast cancer: a short review. Am J Clin Oncol. 2010;33(6):637–45.
15. Punglia, R.S, et al. Local therapy and survival in breast cancer. N Engl J Med. 2007;356(23):2399–405.
16. Haffty BG, et al. Locoregional relapse and distant metastasis in conservatively managed triple negative early-stage breast cancer. J Clin Oncol. 2006;24(36):5652–7.
17. Nguyen PL, et al. Breast cancer subtype approximated by estrogen receptor, progesterone receptor, and HER-2 is associated with local and distant recurrence after breast-conserving therapy. J Clin Oncol. 2008;26(14):2373–8.
18. Millar EK, et al. Prediction of local recurrence, distant metastases, and death after breast-conserving therapy in early-stage invasive breast cancer using a five-biomarker panel. J Clin Oncol. 2009;27(28):4701–8.
19. Lowery AJ, et al. Locoregional recurrence after breast cancer surgery: a systematic review by receptor phenotype. Breast Cancer Res Treat. 2012;133(3):831–41.
20. Abdulkarim BS, et al. Increased risk of locoregional recurrence for women with T1-2N0 triple-negative breast cancer treated with modified radical mastectomy without adjuvant radiation therapy compared with breast-conserving therapy. J Clin Oncol. 2011;29(21):2852–8.
21. Kindts I, et al. Omitting radiation therapy in women with triple-negative breast cancer leads to worse breast cancer-specific survival. The Breast. 32:18–25.
22. Moran MS, et al. Society of Surgical Oncology–American Society for Radiation Oncology Consensus Guideline on Margins for Breast-Conserving Surgery with Whole-Breast Irradiation in Stages I and II Invasive Breast Cancer. Ann Surg Oncol. 2014;21(3):704–16.
23. Pilewskie M, et al. Effect of margin width on local recurrence in triple-negative breast cancer patients treated with breast-conserving therapy. Ann Surg Oncol. 2014;21(4):1209–14.
24. Punglia RS, et al. Impact of interval from breast conserving surgery to radiotherapy on local recurrence in older women with breast cancer: retrospective cohort analysis. BMJ. 2010;340
25. Huang J, et al. Does delay in starting treatment affect the outcomes of radiotherapy? A systematic review. J Clin Oncol. 2003;21(3):555–63.
26. Gupta S, et al. The effect of waiting times for postoperative radiotherapy on outcomes for women receiving partial mastectomy for breast cancer: a systematic review and meta-analysis. Clinical Oncology. 28(12):739–49.

27. Vrieling C, et al. Prognostic factors for local control in breast cancer after long-term fol-
    low-up in the EORTC boost vs no boost trial: a randomized clinical trial. JAMA Oncol.
    2017;3(1):42–8.
28. Bartelink H, et al. Whole-breast irradiation with or without a boost for patients treated with
    breast-conserving surgery for early breast cancer: 20-year follow-up of a randomised phase 3
    trial. Lancet Oncol. 2015;16(1):47–56.
29. Offersen BV, et al. ESTRO consensus guideline on target volume delineation for elective radi-
    ation therapy of early stage breast cancer. Radiother Oncol. 2015;114(1):3–10.
30. The S.T.G, et al. The UK Standardisation of Breast Radiotherapy (START) TTrial B of radio-
    therapy hypofractionation for treatment of early breast cancer: a randomised trial. Lancet.
    371(9618):1098–107.
31. Whelan TJ, et al. Long-term results of hypofractionated radiation therapy for breast cancer. N
    Engl J Med. 2010;362(6):513–20.
32. Hypofractionated radiotherapy for breast cancer. N Engl J Med. 2010;362(19):1843–4.
33. Bane AL, et al. Tumor factors predictive of response to hypofractionated radiotherapy in a
    randomized trial following breast conserving therapy. Ann Oncol. 2014;25(5):992–8.
34. Smith BD, et al. Fractionation for whole breast irradiation: an American Society for
    Radiation Oncology (ASTRO) evidence-based guideline. Int J Radiat Oncol Biol Phys.
    2011;81(1):59–68.
35. Anderson BM, et al. Locoregional recurrence by molecular subtype after multicatheter inter-
    stitial accelerated partial breast irradiation: results from the Pooled Registry of Multicatheter
    Interstitial Sites research group. Brachytherapy. 2016;15(6):788–95.
36. Wilkinson JB, et al. Outcomes according to breast cancer subtype in patients treated with
    accelerated partial breast irradiation. Clin Breast Cancer. 2017;17(1):55–60.
37. Strnad V, et al. 5-year results of accelerated partial breast irradiation using sole interstitial
    multicatheter brachytherapy versus whole-breast irradiation with boost after breast-conserving
    surgery for low-risk invasive and in-situ carcinoma of the female breast: a randomised, phase
    3, non-inferiority trial. Lancet. 387(10015):229–38.
38. Ferlay J, et al. Estimates of worldwide burden of cancer in 2008: GLOBOCAN 2008. Int J
    Cancer. 2010;127(12):2893–917.
39. Konigsberg R, et al. Breast cancer subtypes in patients aged 70 years and older. Cancer Invest.
    2016;34(5):197–204.
40. Wildiers H, et al. Relationship between age and axillary lymph node involvement in women
    with breast cancer. J Clin Oncol. 2009;27(18):2931–7.
41. Bastiaannet E, et al. Lack of survival gain for elderly women with breast cancer. Oncologist.
    2011;16(4):415–23.
42. Barthelemy P, et al. Adjuvant chemotherapy in elderly patients with early breast cancer. Impact
    of age and comprehensive geriatric assessment on tumor board proposals. Crit Rev Oncol
    Hematol. 2011;79(2):196–204.
43. Lin NU, et al. Clinicopathologic features, patterns of recurrence, and survival among women
    with triple-negative breast cancer in the National Comprehensive Cancer Network. Cancer.
    2012;118(22):5463–72.
44. Gangi A, et al. Triple-negative breast cancer is not associated with increased likelihood of
    nodal metastases. Ann Surg Oncol. 2014;21(13):4098–103.
45. Giuliano AE, et al. Locoregional recurrence after sentinel lymph node dissection with or with-
    out axillary dissection in patients with sentinel lymph node metastases: long-term follow-
    up from the American College of Surgeons Oncology Group (Alliance) ACOSOG Z0011
    Randomized Trial. Ann Surg. 2016;264(3):413–20.
46. Donker M, et al. Radiotherapy or surgery of the axilla after a positive sentinel node in breast
    cancer (EORTC 10981-22023 AMAROS): a randomised, multicentre, open-label, phase 3
    non-inferiority trial. Lancet Oncol. 2014;15(12):1303–10.
47. Hennequin C, et al. Ten-year survival results of a randomized trial of irradiation of internal
    mammary nodes after mastectomy. Int J Radiat Oncol Biol Phys. 2013;86(5):860–6.
48. Whelan TJ, et al. Regional nodal irradiation in early-stage breast cancer. N Engl J Med.
    2015;373(4):307–16.

49. Poortmans PM, et al. Internal mammary and medial supraclavicular irradiation in breast cancer. N Engl J Med. 2015;373(4):317–27.
50. Liedtke C, et al. Response to neoadjuvant therapy and long-term survival in patients with triple-negative breast cancer. J Clin Oncol. 2008;26(8):1275–81.
51. Jwa E, et al. Locoregional recurrence by tumor biology in breast cancer patients after preoperative chemotherapy and breast conservation treatment. Cancer Res Treat. 2016;48(4):1363–72.
52. Mamounas EP, et al. Predictors of locoregional recurrence after neoadjuvant chemotherapy: results from combined analysis of National Surgical Adjuvant Breast and Bowel Project B-18 and B-27. J Clin Oncol. 2012;30(32):3960–6.
53. Kyndi M, et al. Estrogen receptor, progesterone receptor, HER-2, and response to postmastectomy radiotherapy in high-risk breast cancer: the Danish Breast Cancer Cooperative Group. J Clin Oncol. 2008;26(9):1419–26.
54. Kyndi M, et al. High local recurrence risk is not associated with large survival reduction after postmastectomy radiotherapy in high-risk breast cancer: a subgroup analysis of DBCG 82 b&c. Radiother Oncol. 2009;90(1):74–9.
55. O'Rorke MA, et al. The value of adjuvant radiotherapy on survival and recurrence in triple-negative breast cancer: a systematic review and meta-analysis of 5507 patients. Cancer Treat Rev. 47:12–21.
56. Truong PT, et al. Is biological subtype prognostic of locoregional recurrence risk in women with pT1-2N0 breast cancer treated with mastectomy? Int J Radiat Oncol Biol Phys. 2014;88(1):57–64.
57. Chen X, et al. Radiotherapy can improve the disease-free survival rate in triple-negative breast cancer patients with T1-T2 disease and one to three positive lymph nodes after mastectomy. Oncologist. 2013;18(2):141–7.
58. Wang J, et al. Adjuvant chemotherapy and radiotherapy in triple-negative breast carcinoma: a prospective randomized controlled multi-center trial. Radiother Oncol. 2011;100(2):200–4.

Optimizing Adjuvant and Neoadjuvant Chemotherapy for Triple-Negative Breast Cancer

7

Sonya Reid-Lawrence, Antoinette R. Tan, and Ingrid A. Mayer

Clinical Pearls
- Anthracycline-, alkylator-, and taxane-based chemotherapy are the current standard treatment regimens for a high-risk, early-stage, and locally advanced triple-negative breast cancer.
- For low-risk, small, node-negative triple-negative tumors, consider shorter regimens such as doxorubicin and cyclophosphamide (AC), docetaxel and cyclophosphamide (TC), or cyclophosphamide, methotrexate, and 5-fluorouracil (CMF).
- For BRCA-mutated triple-negative breast cancer, consider addition of platinum in the neoadjuvant setting.
- For TNBC patients who do not achieve a pathologic complete response after neoadjuvant chemotherapy, consider the use of adjuvant capecitabine or clinical trial enrollment.

7.1   Introduction

Triple-negative breast cancer (TNBC) is defined as the absence of estrogen receptor (ER) and progesterone receptor (PR) and lack of amplification of the human epidermal growth factor receptor type 2 (HER2). TNBC accounts for approximately 15–20% of all invasive breast cancers. Most TNBCs are high-grade, and

S. Reid-Lawrence, MBBS • I.A. Mayer, MD, MSCI (✉)
Division of Hematology/Oncology, Vanderbilt University Medical Center,
Vanderbilt-Ingram Cancer Center, Nashville, TN, USA
e-mail: sonya.a.reid-lawrence@vanderbilt.edu; ingrid.mayer@vanderbilt.edu

A.R. Tan, MD, MHSc, FACP
Department of Solid Tumor Oncology and Investigational Therapeutics,
Levine Cancer Institute, Carolinas HealthCare System, Charlotte, NC, USA
e-mail: antoinette.tan@carolinashealthcare.org

© Springer International Publishing AG 2018
A.R. Tan (ed.), *Triple-Negative Breast Cancer*,
https://doi.org/10.1007/978-3-319-69980-6_7

the majority of them harbor a basal-like gene expression signature [1]. TNBCs are known to be an aggressive group of breast cancers with higher rates of relapse stage for stage compared to ER−/PR-positive and HER2-amplified breast cancers [2]. The mainstay of treatment for TNBC is cytotoxic chemotherapy. Despite the heterogeneous nature of the disease and no known targetable biomarker, TNBC has higher response rates to neoadjuvant chemotherapy compared to other breast cancer subtypes, which is referred to as the TNBC paradox [3]. In this chapter, we will review the treatment strategies utilized in the adjuvant and neoadjuvant settings for TNBC.

7.2 Adjuvant Chemotherapy Considerations for Triple-Negative Breast Cancer

The adjuvant therapy of breast cancer has resulted in significant disease-free survival (DFS) and overall survival (OS) benefits for those affected. At present, chemotherapy is the main approach for the adjuvant treatment of TNBC. There have been many retrospective studies that have evaluated different adjuvant chemotherapy regimens, but not all have been specific to the triple-negative subset, mainly because of minimal available information on HER2 status when these analyses were conducted.

The Early Breast Cancer Trialists' Collaborative Group demonstrated that the use of polychemotherapy in the adjuvant setting conferred a significant reduction in recurrent disease and mortality from breast cancer and also all-cause mortality in ER-negative or ER-poor breast cancer [4]. In another meta-analysis, ER-negative, node-positive breast cancer patients had improved OS by 16.7% compared to 4% for the ER-positive counterpart [5]. From these data, it can be inferred that adjuvant chemotherapy has had a significant impact on the outcome of patients with TNBC.

7.3 Adjuvant Versus Neoadjuvant Therapy for Triple-Negative Breast Cancer

Due to a variety of reasons, initial surgery followed by the use of adjuvant chemotherapy may be the predominant practice or the preferred option compared to preoperative or neoadjuvant chemotherapy for a particular patient [6]. It is reported that chemotherapy use in the neoadjuvant and adjuvant settings generally provides the same long-term outcome [7]. Neoadjuvant therapy is often considered in the management of TNBC. The advantages include downstaging tumor size to allow for breast-conservative surgery in selected cases, limiting the extent of axillary node sampling, rendering an inoperable tumor operable, and obtaining an in vivo assessment of tumor sensitivity to chemotherapy.

Despite optimal systemic chemotherapy, only 30% of women treated with standard neoadjuvant anthracycline and taxane-based chemotherapy will achieve a pathological complete response (pCR), defined as lack of residual disease in both the breast and axilla [8]. It is generally established that patients with breast cancer who achieve a pCR after neoadjuvant therapy exhibit good long-term outcome [9]. More specifically, approximately 30% of TNBCs treated with anthracycline- and taxane-based neoadjuvant chemotherapy have a pCR to treatment, and consistent with above data, achieving a pCR to neoadjuvant chemotherapy in this group of patients also has been shown to be a strongly positive prognostic factor [8]. On the other hand, those patients with residual viable tumor following neoadjuvant therapy are at risk for metastatic recurrence and death [10, 11].

7.4 Adjuvant Regimens for Triple-Negative Breast Cancer

To reduce the risk of recurrent disease in a patient with TNBC after definitive surgery, the standard adjuvant therapy consists of a regimen that contains an anthracycline, an alkylator, and a taxane. There are several commonly used adjuvant regimens endorsed by several organizations including the American Society of Clinical Oncology (ASCO) and the National Comprehensive Cancer Network (NCCN) for HER-negative disease, and its use can be extrapolated to the treatment of TNBCs (Table 7.1) [12, 13]. In general, adjuvant chemotherapy is recommended in a TNBC patient with lymph node-positive disease (N1 or greater), regardless of primary tumor size, and in node-negative disease that is greater than 1 cm. These regimens are also often utilized interchangeably in the neoadjuvant setting.

Several studies, including National Surgical Adjuvant Breast and Bowel Project (NSABP) B-30 and Eastern Cooperative Oncology Group (ECOG) 1199, have shown the benefit of sequential administration of anthracycline and taxane in

Table 7.1 Commonly used regimens in the adjuvant and neoadjuvant settings for high-risk triple-negative breast cancer

Sequential
• Doxorubicin-cyclophosphamide × 4 → paclitaxel administered once per week × 12 weeks
Doxorubicin 60 mg/m² IV day 1
Cyclophosphamide 600 mg/m² IV day 1
Cycled every 21 days for four cycles
Followed by:
Paclitaxel 80 mg/m² IV weekly for 12 weeks
• Dose-dense doxorubicin-cyclophosphamide × 4 → dose-dense paclitaxel × 4
Doxorubicin 60 mg/m² IV day 1
Cyclophosphamide 600 mg/m² IV day 1
Cycled every 14 days for four cycles with myeloid growth factor support
Followed by:
Paclitaxel 175 mg/m² IV day 1
Cycled every 14 days for four cycles with myeloid growth factor support

(continued)

Table 7.1 (continued)

• Doxorubicin-cyclophosphamide × 4 → docetaxel × 4
Doxorubicin 60 mg/m^2 IV day 1
Cyclophosphamide 600 mg/m^2 IV day 1
Cycled every 21 days for four cycles
Followed by:
Docetaxel 100 mg/m^2 IV day 1
Cycled every 21 days for four cycles
• Fluorouracil-epirubicin-cyclophosphamide × 3 → docetaxel × 3
Fluorouracil 500 mg/m^2 IV day 1
Epirubicin 100 mg/m^2 IV day 1
Cyclophosphamide 500 mg/m^2 IV day 1
Cycled every 21 days for three cycles
Followed by:
Docetaxel 100 mg/m^2 IV day 1
Cycled every 21 days for three cycles
• Dose-dense epirubicin-cyclophosphamide × four cycles → dose-dense paclitaxel × four cycles
Epirubicin 90 mg/m^2 IV day 1
Cyclophosphamide 600 mg/m^2 IV day 1
Cycled every 14 days for four cycles with myeloid growth factor support
Followed by:
Paclitaxel 175 mg/m^2 IV day 1
Cycled every 14 days for four cycles with myeloid growth factor support
Concurrent
• Docetaxel-doxorubicin-cyclophosphamide × 6
Docetaxel 75 mg/m^2 IV day 1
Doxorubicin 50 mg/m^2 IV day 1
Cyclophosphamide 500 mg/m^2 IV day 1
Cycled every 21 days for six cycles; can give with myeloid growth factor support
Non-anthracycline-containing regimens
• Docetaxel-cyclophosphamide × 4
Docetaxel 75 mg/m^2 IV day 1
Cyclophosphamide 600 mg/m^2 IV day 1
Cycled every 21 days for four cycles with myeloid growth factor support
• Docetaxel-carboplatin × 6
Docetaxel 75 mg/m^2 IV day 1
Carboplatin AUC 6 IV day 1
Cycled every 21 days for six cycles with myeloid growth factor support
• Cyclophosphamide-methotrexate-fluorouracil × 6
Cyclophosphamide 100 mg/m^2 PO days 1–14
Methotrexate 40 mg/m^2 IV days 1 and 8
Fluorouracil 600 mg/m^2 IV days 1 and 8
Cycled every 28 days for six cycles

ER-negative breast cancer (Table 7.2) [14, 15]. The addition of taxanes sequentially in the treatment of early-stage HER2-negative breast cancer has been demonstrated in other studies including the Cancer Leukemia Group B (CALGB) 9344/INT1048 study, which compared doxorubicin and cyclophosphamide (AC) ± paclitaxel, and GEICAM 9906 study, which compared 5-fluorouracil, epirubicin, and

Table 7.2 Select adjuvant clinical trials evaluating taxanes in breast cancer

Study	N	LN+ (%)	Timing of taxane	Arms	5-year DFS (%)	5-year OS (%)
ECOG 1199	4950	88	Sequential	Tw × 12	78	86
				T × 4	81	87
				Pw × 12	82	90
				P × 4	77	87
CALGB 9344/ INT1048	3121	100	Sequential	AC × 4	65	77
				AC × 4 → P × 4	70	80
GEICAM 9906	1246	100	Sequential	FEC × 6	72	87
				FEC × 4 → Pw × 8	79	90
BCIRG 001	1491	100	Concurrent	FAC × 6	68	81
				TAC × 6	75	87
GEICAM 9805	1059	0	Concurrent	FAC × 6	86	95
				TAC × 6	91	97
NSABP B-38	4894	100	Concurrent and sequential	TAC × 6	80	90
				ddAC x 4 → ddP × 4	82	89
				ddAC × 4 → ddPG × 4	81	91

Abbreviations: *AC* doxorubicin and cyclophosphamide every 3 weeks; *BCIRG* Breast Cancer International Research Group; *CALGB* Cancer and Leukemia Group B; *ddAC* dose-dense doxorubicin and cyclophosphamide every 2 weeks; *DFS* disease-free survival; *ddP* dose-dense paclitaxel every 2 weeks; *ddPG* dose-dense paclitaxel and gemcitabine every 2 weeks; *ECOG* Eastern Cooperative Oncology Group; *LN+* percentage of patients with axillary lymph node involvement; *FAC* fluorouracil, doxorubicin, and cyclophosphamide; *FEC* fluorouracil, epirubicin, and cyclophosphamide; *N* number of patients; *NSABP* National Surgical Adjuvant Breast and Bowel Project; *OS* overall survival; *P* paclitaxel every 3 weeks; *Pw* paclitaxel weekly; *T* docetaxel every 3 weeks; *TAC* docetaxel, doxorubicin, and cyclophosphamide; *Tw* docetaxel weekly

cyclophosphamide (FEC) ± paclitaxel [16, 17]. In these studies, subset analyses showed that the addition of taxanes benefited TNBC. In addition, the concurrent use of a taxane with an anthracycline and cyclophosphamide has been shown to be more effective than a combination without it. The Breast Cancer International Research Group (BCIRG) 001 adjuvant trial demonstrated that docetaxel, doxorubicin, and cyclophosphamide (TAC) resulted in improved DFS and OS compared to 5-fluorouracil, doxorubicin, and cyclophosphamide (FAC) in the TNBC node-positive subset [18, 19]. The GEICAM 9805 study demonstrated that TAC was better than FAC in the adjuvant therapy of high-risk node-negative breast cancer and in the TNBC subgroup [20]. The use of taxanes sequentially or concomitantly is acceptable. In the large adjuvant NSABP B-38 study, the combination of TAC did not show a benefit compared to the dose-dense sequential format with AC followed by paclitaxel, and the toxicity profile of each regimen differed [21].

There is also evidence that administration of paclitaxel weekly for 12 doses compared to docetaxel every 3 weeks or paclitaxel every 3 weeks for 4 doses, following 4 cycles of AC in the adjuvant setting, leads to improved DFS and OS in the triple-negative subset [15]. Another common schedule that is used in the adjuvant setting is the dose-dense sequential regimen in which paclitaxel is given every 2 weeks with growth factor support. The Southwestern Oncology Group (SWOG) S0221 study showed there was no difference in efficacy comparing the dose-dense therapy of every 2 weeks with weekly paclitaxel in the TNBC subgroup and superiority of delivering paclitaxel every 2 weeks compared to every 3 weeks [22].

Numerous strategies have been tested to enhance the current standard approaches to reduce the risk of recurrence of early-stage TNBC. NSABP B-38 did not show any benefit of adding a fourth drug, gemcitabine, to an anthracycline and taxane sequence in the adjuvant treatment of node-positive, HER2-negative breast cancer [21]. The targeted agent, bevacizumab, a monoclonal antibody to vascular endothelial growth factor A, when added to standard adjuvant chemotherapy in early-stage TNBC did not result in an improvement in OS in the BEATRICE trial [23]. The role of carboplatin is being evaluated in the NRG-BR003 phase III adjuvant clinical trial in which high-risk early-stage TNBC patients are randomized to AC followed by paclitaxel with or without carboplatin (NCT02488967).

In summary, a sequential dose-dense AC and dose-dense paclitaxel regimen and a sequential anthracycline/alkylator followed by a weekly taxane are often-used approaches to treat an early-stage TNBC patient. A concurrent anthracycline, alkylator, and taxane combination is also deemed acceptable. In some countries, an epirubicin-based regimen consisting of epirubicin and cyclophosphamide ± fluorouracil followed by a taxane is considered standard treatment for a patient with early-stage TNBC [24].

7.5   Small Node-Negative Triple-Negative Breast Cancers

Exceptions to administering a multidrug backbone regimen include extremely small triple-negative breast tumors and patients who are not eligible to receive anthracyclines or taxanes. For a T1aN0 or T1bN0 triple-negative tumor (≤ 1 cm), there is minimal information available regarding the benefit of chemotherapy and what the optimal chemotherapy regimen is. Clinicians need to discuss the risk/benefit ratio when faced with a patient with a triple-negative tumor that is 1 cm or less. A retrospective study from a single institution reported on the outcome of 194 node-negative, triple-negative patients with tumors 1 cm or less and found they had a favorable prognosis, with a 5-year distant recurrence-free survival rate of 95% and no difference whether they were treated with chemotherapy or not [25].

Another issue with regard to these small node-negative, triple-negative tumors is whether a non-anthracycline chemotherapy regimen can be given. The ASCO guidelines offer some guidance on adjuvant regimens when an anthracycline is not preferred or possible, and this could be applied to T1b tumors and certain T1c tumors [12]. The US Oncology Research (USOR) Trial 9735 showed that four cycles of docetaxel and cyclophosphamide (TC) resulted in higher DFS compared to four cycles of AC [26]. Additionally, for patients who are not candidates for treatment with anthracyclines and taxanes, consideration can be given to the combination of cyclophosphamide, methotrexate, and fluorouracil (CMF) for six cycles. In retrospective analyses of adjuvant chemotherapy trials using CMF, the

CMF regimen was shown to have activity in the triple-negative early breast cancer setting [27, 28].

Understanding that the 5-year risk of recurrence of a small, node-negative TNBC is low (less than 10%) with a small treatment benefit, a reasonable algorithm for adjuvant treatment of a node-negative TNBC is to offer chemotherapy if the tumor size is >1 cm (T1c) and otherwise medically appropriate. For triple-negative tumors measuring 0.6–1 cm (T1b), consider chemotherapy and have a balanced discussion with the patient about the benefit and risks. For triple-negative breast cancers 0.5 cm or less (T1a), consider observation.

7.6 Role of Anthracyclines in the Treatment of Triple-Negative Breast Cancer

As previously discussed, one study demonstrates the superiority of TC to AC in the treatment of early-stage HER2-negative breast cancers [26]. In addition, the activity of TC compared to AC regimens with a taxane (AC-Tax) was reported by Harbeck and colleagues which showed that six cycles of TC were not inferior to an AC-Tax regimen in patients with ER+ breast cancers and intermediate-risk TNBC [29]. However, the ABC (anthracycline in early breast cancer) phase III adjuvant trials comparing TC versus TaxAC in 4130 women with resected high-risk, HER2-negative breast cancer showed improved invasive disease-free survival (IDFS) with the addition of anthracycline (86.6% for TC vs. 89.6% for TaxAC with a hazard ratio of 1.42 [1.04–1.94]) [30]. These data suggest that for women with lower risk of recurrence (ER+ breast cancer with up to three involved lymph nodes) and lower-risk TNBC (< T2 N0 tumors), it is reasonable to consider four to six cycles of TC as adjuvant chemotherapy, whereas for women with high-risk HER2-negative breast cancers (≥T2 N0 TNBCs, high-grade ER+ breast cancers with involved lymph nodes), the incorporation of anthracyclines still matters.

7.7 Role of Platinum in the Neoadjuvant Treatment of Triple-Negative Breast Cancer

A large proportion of TNBC would be classified as "basal-like" using gene expression profiling, based on the PAM50 intrinsic subtype classification [31, 32]. These basal-like TNBCs have many similarities to tumors arising in *BRCA1* mutation carriers, including a greater likelihood of being high-grade, ER-negative, PR-negative, and HER2-negative, having high frequency of p53 mutations and expression of basal keratins and clustering together by gene expression profile [33]. Since *BRCA1*-mutated cancers have genomic instability and sensitivity to DNA-cross-linking agents, agents targeted toward DNA repair defects, such as PARP inhibitors and platinum agents, are clinically effective against these tumors [34–36]. These observations generated enthusiasm to evaluate the potential benefit of platinum-based chemotherapy in TNBC.

Several clinical studies have examined the role of platinum analogues such as carboplatin and cisplatin in the neoadjuvant treatment of TNBC. These studies utilized rates of pCR as an endpoint, since it is generally accepted that patients who achieve a higher pCR exhibit improved long-term outcomes, while a high residual disease burden post-neoadjuvant chemotherapy correlates with a high rate of recurrence and death [8, 9]. In a study conducted in Poland by Byrski and colleagues, a pCR of 61% (65 of 107) was achieved in patients with stage I–III breast cancer with a *BRCA1* mutation after neoadjuvant therapy with four cycles of cisplatin [37]. In a small single-arm study of 28 women with stage II and III TNBC treated with 4 cycles of neoadjuvant single-agent cisplatin, there was a 22% pCR rate (6 of 28), including 2 patients with *BRCA1* germline mutations; 64% (18 of 28) experienced a clinical complete response (50%) or partial response (14%) [38]. Another trial of 51 early-stage TNBC patients treated with neoadjuvant cisplatin for 4 cycles and bevacizumab for 3 cycles prior to surgery reported a pCR of 15% [39]. The observed single-agent clinical activity of platinum in early-stage TNBC supports its evaluation into our standard neoadjuvant regimens. The results of the INFORM trial (NCT01670500) which is a randomized phase II study of neoadjuvant cisplatin compared to AC in newly diagnosed breast cancer with germline *BRCA* mutations should add additional important insight on the role of platinum in our clinical management of TNBC.

GeparSixto and CALGB 40603 are two large randomized phase II neoadjuvant trials that evaluated the effect of platinum-based agents in TNBC with similar designs. The GeparSixto phase II trial from the German Breast Group compared a weekly paclitaxel and nonpegylated liposomal doxorubicin × 18 weeks and every 3-week bevacizumab regimen with or without weekly carboplatin in 315 early-stage TNBC patients [40]. In this study, the addition of carboplatin increased the pCR rate in the breast and axillary lymph nodes from 37% to 53% ($P = 0.005$). The CALGB 40603 (Alliance) phase II trial evaluated the impact of adding 4 cycles of carboplatin every 3 weeks and/or bevacizumab to neoadjuvant weekly paclitaxel × 12 followed by 4 cycles of dose-dense doxorubicin and cyclophosphamide (ddAC) in 443 stage II or III TNBC patients [41]. In this study, the addition of carboplatin significantly increased the rate of pCR in the breast and lymph nodes from approximately 41% to 54% ($P = 0.0029$). There was an improvement in 3-year event-free survival (EFS) in the GeparSixto trial from 76.1% to 85.8% (hazard ratio, 0.56; $P = 0.035$); however, the CALGB 40603 did not show any improvement in EFS. It is important to note that neither study was powered to address EFS or OS benefit from the addition of carboplatin to neoadjuvant chemotherapy. Lack of precision from small sample sizes is likely responsible for the difference seen in DFS in these two trials [42]. There is also not a confirmed correlation between increased rate of pCR and EFS. A pooled analysis by Cortazar and colleagues could not validate pCR as a surrogate endpoint for improved EFS and OS as some patients who achieve a pCR go onto relapse and many with residual disease never experience a recurrence, and small differences in pCR may never translate to improvements in EFS [43]. The improvement in pCR rates in both of these trials came at the expense of increased toxicity with approximately 50% of patients undergoing dose omissions or reductions.

In the setting of a patient with early-stage TNBC who is not a candidate for anthracycline secondary to cardiac dysfunction or has reached a prior maximum lifetime dosage of anthracycline, there are several small studies that have evaluated an anthracycline-free platinum/taxane regimen in the neoadjuvant setting. Sharma and colleagues demonstrated that a pCR rate of 59% and 56% can be achieved in stage I–III TNBC, BRCA-mutated and BRCA wild-type, respectively, after neoadjuvant treatment with docetaxel and carboplatin every 3 weeks × 6 cycles [44]. This would be a reasonable regimen to consider giving in this subset of TNBC patients.

In summary, the addition of platinum agents to the neoadjuvant treatment of TNBC is most compelling in the setting of a young patient with a high-risk BRCA-mutated triple-negative tumor, but it may be reasonable for patients in whom an increase in clinical response to systemic treatment could improve locoregional control (i.e., patients with inflammatory breast cancer or inoperable TNBC at the time of diagnosis). In unselected patients, the utility of platinum agents added to standard neoadjuvant chemotherapy remains controversial as it is unclear whether it improves long-term outcomes.

7.8   Post-Neoadjuvant Setting

Upon completion of neoadjuvant therapy and surgery, the standard of care for patients with TNBC who have no clinical evidence of metastatic disease after surgical excision of the cancer regardless of burden of residual disease is observation. However, patients with TNBC who have a high amount of residual disease, after completing neoadjuvant therapy, have a very high risk of recurrence. The question of whether additional chemotherapy will benefit TNBC with residual disease after completion of neoadjuvant chemotherapy will be answered fully with data from three post-neoadjuvant trials, which include CREATE-X, EA1131, and S1418.

The Japanese phase III CREATE-X (JBCRG-04) trial randomized 910 Asian patients with stage I–IIIB HER2-negative breast cancer with a lack of pCR post-neoadjuvant chemotherapy containing anthracycline, taxane, or both to observation or capecitabine for up to eight cycles [45]. Capecitabine was given at a dose of 2500 mg/m^2/day in two divided doses orally per day on days 1–14 every 3 weeks. In a preplanned subset analysis, among patients with TNBC, the rate of DFS was 69.8% in the capecitabine group versus 56.1% in the control group (hazard ratio for recurrence, second cancer, or death, 0.58; 95% CI, 0.39–0.87), and the OS rate was 78.8% versus 70.3% (hazard ratio for death, 0.52; 95% CI, 0.30–0.90), yielding an absolute OS advantage of almost 9% for those treated with capecitabine.

The other two large studies in the post-neoadjuvant setting specifically in TNBC patients with residual disease in the breast and nodes after neoadjuvant chemotherapy are ongoing. A phase III randomized trial EA1131 (NCT02445391) from the Eastern Cooperative Oncology Group-American College of Radiology Imaging Network (ECOG-ACRIN) will evaluate which subset of TNBC patients with residual disease post-completion of neoadjuvant anthracycline/taxane chemotherapy will have an improved DFS with addition of cisplatin or carboplatin versus capecitabine. The results of this trial will ultimately help avoid exposing up front unselected patients, many of whom will never relapse, to toxic therapy in the absence of long-term known benefit. S1418 (NRG-BR006, NCT02954874) is another randomized phase III clinical trial evaluating the efficacy and safety of pembrolizumab for 1 year, an antibody directed at programmed cell death receptor 1, versus observation as adjuvant therapy for patients with TNBC residual invasive disease after neoadjuvant chemotherapy. Though CREATE-X yielded positive results, it is a single trial. At this time, it is reasonable to discuss the role of capecitabine in patients who meet the eligibility criteria for the CREATE-X trial or to consider enrollment onto a clinical trial. Of note, there are known pharmacokinetic and pharmacogenomic differences in the metabolism of capecitabine that explain why an Asian population can tolerate a higher oral dose of capecitabine [46]. One can consider giving a starting dose of capecitabine at 2000 mg/m^2/day in divided doses on days 1–14 every 3 weeks and adjust based on tolerance.

Conclusion

TNBC is a heterogeneous and complex disease. Neoadjuvant and adjuvant anthracycline-, alkylator-, and taxane-based chemotherapy are the standard backbone regimens for high-risk TNBC. Small, subcentimeter triple-negative tumors can be treated with shorter-course chemotherapy. The addition of a platinum agent routinely in the neoadjuvant setting in TNBC is still an individualized decision and not yet standard of care for all patients. The use of additional cytotoxic agents in triple-negative patients with residual disease post-neoadjuvant chemotherapy will depend on results of ongoing trials. Several clinical trial efforts are in progress to evaluate novel strategies with the hope of improving outcomes for TNBC.

References

1. Dent R, Trudeau M, Pritchard KI, et al. Triple-negative breast cancer: clinical features and patterns of recurrence. Clin Cancer Res. 2007;13:4429–34.
2. Millikan RC, Newman B, Tse CK, et al. Epidemiology of basal-like breast cancer. Breast Cancer Res Treat. 2008;109:123–39.
3. Carey LA, Dees EC, Sawyer L, et al. The triple negative paradox: primary tumor chemosensitivity of breast cancer subtypes. Clin Cancer Res. 2007;13:2329–34.
4. Early Breast Cancer Trialists' Collaborative G, Clarke M, Coates AS, et al. Adjuvant chemotherapy in oestrogen-receptor-poor breast cancer: patient-level meta-analysis of randomised trials. Lancet. 2008;371:29–40.
5. Berry DA, Cirrincione C, Henderson IC, et al. Estrogen-receptor status and outcomes of modern chemotherapy for patients with node-positive breast cancer. JAMA. 2006;295:1658–67.
6. Killelea BK, Yang VQ, Mougalian S, et al. Neoadjuvant chemotherapy for breast cancer increases the rate of breast conservation: results from the national cancer database. J Am Coll Surg. 2015;220:1063–9.
7. Rastogi P, Anderson SJ, Bear HD, et al. Preoperative chemotherapy: updates of National Surgical Adjuvant Breast and bowel project protocols B-18 and B-27. J Clin Oncol. 2008;26:778–85.

8. von Minckwitz G, Untch M, Blohmer JU, et al. Definition and impact of pathologic complete response on prognosis after neoadjuvant chemotherapy in various intrinsic breast cancer subtypes. J Clin Oncol. 2012;30:1796–804.
9. Liedtke C, Mazouni C, Hess KR, et al. Response to neoadjuvant therapy and long-term survival in patients with triple-negative breast cancer. J Clin Oncol. 2008;26:1275–81.
10. Jones RL, Salter J, A'Hern R, et al. The prognostic significance of Ki67 before and after neoadjuvant chemotherapy in breast cancer. Breast Cancer Res Treat. 2009;116:53–68.
11. Guarneri V, Piacentini F, Ficarra G, et al. A prognostic model based on nodal status and Ki-67 predicts the risk of recurrence and death in breast cancer patients with residual disease after preoperative chemotherapy. Ann Oncol. 2009;20:1193–8.
12. Denduluri N, Somerfield MR, Eisen A, et al. Selection of optimal adjuvant chemotherapy regimens for human epidermal growth factor receptor 2 (HER2)-negative and adjuvant targeted therapy for HER2-positive breast cancers: an American Society of Clinical Oncology guideline adaptation of the cancer care Ontario clinical practice guideline. J Clin Oncol. 2016;34:2416–27.
13. National Comprehensive Cancer Network. Breast cancer (Version 2.2017-April 6, 2017). https://www.nccn.org/professionals/physician_gls/pdf/breast.pdf. Accessed 27 Aug 2017.
14. Swain SM, Jeong JH, Geyer CE Jr, et al. Longer therapy, iatrogenic amenorrhea, and survival in early breast cancer. N Engl J Med. 2010;362:2053–65.
15. Sparano JA, Zhao F, Martino S, et al. Long-term follow-up of the E1199 phase III trial evaluating the role of taxane and schedule in operable breast cancer. J Clin Oncol. 2015;33:2353–60.
16. Hayes DF, Thor AD, Dressler LG, et al. HER2 and response to paclitaxel in node-positive breast cancer. N Engl J Med. 2007;357:1496–506.
17. Martin M, Rodriguez-Lescure A, Ruiz A, et al. Molecular predictors of efficacy of adjuvant weekly paclitaxel in early breast cancer. Breast Cancer Res Treat. 2010;123:149–57.
18. Martin M, Pienkowski T, Mackey J, et al. Adjuvant docetaxel for node-positive breast cancer. N Engl J Med. 2005;352:2302–13.
19. Hugh J, Hanson J, Cheang MC, et al. Breast cancer subtypes and response to docetaxel in node-positive breast cancer: use of an immunohistochemical definition in the BCIRG 001 trial. J Clin Oncol. 2009;27:1168–76.
20. Martin M, Segui MA, Anton A, et al. Adjuvant docetaxel for high-risk, node-negative breast cancer. N Engl J Med. 2010;363:2200–10.
21. Swain SM, Tang G, Geyer CE Jr, et al. Definitive results of a phase III adjuvant trial comparing three chemotherapy regimens in women with operable, node-positive breast cancer: the NSABP B-38 trial. J Clin Oncol. 2013;31:3197–204.
22. Budd GT, Barlow WE, Moore HC, et al. SWOG S0221: a phase III trial comparing chemotherapy schedules in high-risk early-stage breast cancer. J Clin Oncol. 2015;33:58–64.
23. Bell R, Brown J, Parmar M, et al. Final efficacy and updated safety results of the randomized phase III BEATRICE trial evaluating adjuvant bevacizumab-containing therapy in triple-negative early breast cancer. Ann Oncol. 2017;28:754–60.
24. Martin M, Rodriguez-Lescure A, Ruiz A, et al. Randomized phase 3 trial of fluorouracil, epirubicin, and cyclophosphamide alone or followed by paclitaxel for early breast cancer. J Natl Cancer Inst. 2008;100:805–14.
25. Ho AY, Gupta G, King TA, et al. Favorable prognosis in patients with T1a/T1bN0 triple-negative breast cancers treated with multimodality therapy. Cancer. 2012;118:4944–52.
26. Jones SE, Savin MA, Holmes FA, et al. Phase III trial comparing doxorubicin plus cyclophosphamide with docetaxel plus cyclophosphamide as adjuvant therapy for operable breast cancer. J Clin Oncol. 2006;24:5381–7.
27. Cheang MC, Voduc KD, Tu D, et al. Responsiveness of intrinsic subtypes to adjuvant anthracycline substitution in the NCIC.CTG MA.5 randomized trial. Clin Cancer Res. 2012;18:2402–12.

28. Colleoni M, Cole BF, Viale G, et al. Classical cyclophosphamide, methotrexate, and fluoroura-cil chemotherapy is more effective in triple-negative, node-negative breast cancer: results from two randomized trials of adjuvant chemoendocrine therapy for node-negative breast cancer. J Clin Oncol. 2010;28:2966–73.
29. Harbeck N, Gluz O, Clemens MR, et al. Prospective WSG phase III PlanB trial: Final analysis of adjuvant 4 x EC→4 x docetaxel vs. 6 x docetaxel/cyclophosphamide in patients with high clinical risk and intermediate-to-high genomic risk HER2-negative, early breast cancer. J Clin Oncol. 35 suppl (abstract 504), 2017.
30. Blum JL, Flynn PJ, Yothers G, et al. Anthracyclines in early breast cancer: the ABC trials-USOR 06-090, NSABP B-46-I/USOR 07132, and NSABP B-49 (NRG oncology). J Clin Oncol. 2017;35:2647–55.
31. Perou CM, Sorlie T, Eisen MB, et al. Molecular portraits of human breast tumours. Nature. 2000;406:747–52.
32. Bertucci F, Finetti P, Cervera N, et al. How basal are triple-negative breast cancers? Int J Cancer. 2008;123:236–40.
33. Matros E, Wang ZC, Lodeiro G, et al. BRCA1 promoter methylation in sporadic breast tumors: relationship to gene expression profiles. Breast Cancer Res Treat. 2005;91:179–86.
34. Turner N, Tutt A, Ashworth A. Hallmarks of 'BRCAness' in sporadic cancers. Nat Rev Cancer. 2004;4:814–9.
35. Tutt A, Robson M, Garber JE, et al. Oral poly(ADP-ribose) polymerase inhibitor olaparib in patients with BRCA1 or BRCA2 mutations and advanced breast cancer: a proof-of-concept trial. Lancet. 2010;376:235–44.
36. Byrski T, Huzarski T, Dent R, et al. Response to neoadjuvant therapy with cisplatin in BRCA1-positive breast cancer patients. Breast Cancer Res Treat. 2009;115:359–63.
37. Byrski T, Huzarski T, Dent R, et al. Pathologic complete response to neoadjuvant cisplatin in BRCA1-positive breast cancer patients. Breast Cancer Res Treat. 2014;147:401–5.
38. Silver DP, Richardson AL, Eklund AC, et al. Efficacy of neoadjuvant cisplatin in triple-negative breast cancer. J Clin Oncol. 2010;28:1145–53.
39. Ryan PD, Tung NM, Isakoff SJ, et al. Neoadjuvant cisplatin and bevacizumab in triple-negative breast cancer: Safety and efficacy. J Clin Oncol. 2009;27 suppl (abstract 551).
40. von Minckwitz G, Schneeweiss A, Loibl S, et al. Neoadjuvant carboplatin in patients with triple-negative and HER2-positive early breast cancer (GeparSixto; GBG 66): a randomised phase 2 trial. Lancet Oncol. 2014;15:747–56.
41. Sikov WM, Berry DA, Perou CM, et al. Impact of the addition of carboplatin and/or beva-cizumab to neoadjuvant once-per-week paclitaxel followed by dose-dense doxorubicin and cyclophosphamide on pathologic complete response rates in stage II to III triple-negative breast cancer: CALGB 40603 (alliance). J Clin Oncol. 2015;33:13–21.
42. Prowell TM, Pazdur R. Pathological complete response and accelerated drug approval in early breast cancer. N Engl J Med. 2012;366:2438–41.
43. Cortazar P, Zhang L, Untch M, et al. Pathological complete response and long-term clinical benefit in breast cancer: the CTNeoBC pooled analysis. Lancet. 2014;384:164–72.
44. Sharma P, Lopez-Tarruella S, Garcia-Saenz JA, et al. Efficacy of neoadjuvant carboplatin plus docetaxel in triple-negative breast cancer: combined analysis of two cohorts. Clin Cancer Res. 2017;23:649–57.
45. Masuda N, Lee SJ, Ohtani S, et al. Adjuvant capecitabine for breast cancer after preoperative chemotherapy. N Engl J Med. 2017;376:2147–59.
46. Midgley R, Kerr DJ. Capecitabine: have we got the dose right? Nat Clin Pract Oncol. 2009;6:17–24.

Management of Metastatic Triple-Negative Breast Cancer

Anne P. O'Dea and Priyanka Sharma

Clinical Pearls
- In patients with clinical evidence of metastatic disease, biopsy and reassessment of hormone and human epidermal growth factor receptor type 2 status should be performed.
- Triple-negative breast cancer is characterized by a higher proportion of visceral and soft tissue relapse and lower rates of osseous metastasis, compared to non-triple-negative breast cancer.
- Sequential use of single-agent chemotherapy is the recommended treatment strategy for most patients with metastatic triple-negative breast cancer until progression of disease or significant toxicity.
- Germline *BRCA* status is important in informing a decision for selection of platinum agent in the treatment of metastatic triple-negative breast cancer.
- Participation in clinical trials evaluating novel agents should be encouraged for patients with metastatic triple-negative breast cancer.

8.1   Diagnosis and Clinical Behavior

Diagnosis of TNBC requires ER, PR, and HER2 status testing. Testing and the cut-offs for ER, PR, and HER2 statuses were developed to determine the likelihood of response to endocrine and HER2-directed therapy, respectively, and not to specifically identify the "triple-negative" phenotype. Thus, over the last decade, ER, PR, and HER2 cutoffs used to describe TNBC have varied. Most contemporary studies are now using the current American Society of Clinical Oncology/College of American Pathologists (ASCO/CAP) guidelines for determining ER, PR, and HER2

A.P. O'Dea, MD • P. Sharma, MD (✉)
University of Kansas Medical Center, Westwood, KS, USA
e-mail: aodea@kumc.edu; psharma2@kumc.edu

© Springer International Publishing AG 2018
A.R. Tan (ed.), *Triple-Negative Breast Cancer*,
https://doi.org/10.1007/978-3-319-69980-6_8

negativity (ER and PR nuclear staining of less than 1% by immunohistochemistry (IHC), and HER2 IHC staining 0 to 1+ or FISH ratio < 2.0 if IHC 2+ or IHC not performed) [2, 3].

All patients with clinical evidence of metastatic TNBC should undergo a complete evaluation to assess the extent of their disease. This includes radiographic assessment and confirmatory biopsy of suspected lesions with testing of ER, PR, and HER2 status. Biopsy and reassessment of hormone and HER2 receptor status are recommended by most professional guidelines [2, 8]. This is of significant clinical importance as change in ER or HER2 status has dramatic treatment implications. In an observational study of 184 patients, the rates of discordance in ER, PR, and HER2 status between the primary and recurrent disease were 13%, 28%, and 3%, respectively, leading to alterations of treatment plan (based on phenotype of metastatic disease) in 31% of patients [9]. These findings reinforce the clinical importance of performing confirmatory biopsy of metastases to optimize treatment. Biopsy of extra-osseous site is preferred over biopsy of osseous lesions if deemed feasible and safe. Some studies report that decalcifying agents that enable sectioning of bone may affect protein antigenicity, thus affecting ER, PR, and HER2 assessment [10, 11]. This aspect should be kept in mind when interpreting results of ER, PR, and HER2 status in bone biopsies.

TNBC is associated with not only higher but also earlier risk of relapse. Hazard rates for distant recurrence are highest for TNBC in the first 2 years after diagnosis, and relapses after 5 years are very uncommon [6, 12]. Compared to hormone receptor-positive breast cancer, TNBC is characterized by a higher proportion of visceral and soft tissue relapse and lower rates of osseous metastasis [6, 7]. TNBC patients who develop metastatic disease have a short survival [7, 13]. Median survival of patients with metastatic TNBC is only 12–18 months compared to 5 years for patients with metastatic HER2-positive breast cancer, highlighting the pressing need for identification of more effective systemic therapies for this subgroup [14]. Furthermore, for metastatic TNBC median progression-free survival after first-line chemotherapy is very dismal, about 3–4 months, highlighting the critical need for development of better therapies for treatment of metastatic TNBC [15, 16].

8.2   Triple-Negative Breast Cancer and Germline *BRCA* Mutation

Compared to other subtypes of breast cancers, women with TNBC have a higher prevalence of germline *BRCA* mutations [17–20]. Various studies have demonstrated that 15–20% of women with TNBC carry germline *BRCA 1/2* mutations. Most genetic testing guidelines include TNBC subtype as an independent criterion for hereditary breast and/or ovarian cancer syndrome (HBOC) counseling and testing recommendation. The National Comprehensive Cancer Network (NCCN) guidelines recommend genetic risk assessment of all TNBC patients and HBOC testing for all TNBC patients aged ≤60 years regardless of family history. Despite these recommendations, financial constraints, insurance coverage, and access to genetic counseling and testing continue to be important challenges for optimal utilization of HBOC testing in the clinical setting [19].

8.3 Basic Principles of Treatment

The primary goals of systemic treatment for metastatic breast cancer are prolongation of survival, alleviation or delay of onset of symptoms, and improvement in quality of life. These goals have to be balanced against the toxicity associated with treatment [21–23]. Most general principles that are applied to the treatment of advanced breast cancer of other phenotypes are applicable to TNBC. Due to lack of targeted therapies such as endocrine therapy and anti-HER2 therapy, cytotoxic chemotherapy is still the foundation for systemic treatment of metastatic TNBC. Sequential use of single-agent chemotherapy is the most widely practiced treatment strategy for metastatic TNBC, with the usual approach of treating to either maximal response or intolerable toxicity [22]. Commonly used single chemotherapy agents include taxanes, platinum salts, anthracyclines, antimetabolites, gemcitabine, vinca alkaloids, and non-taxane tubulin polymerizing agents, such as ixabepilone and eribulin (Table 8.1). For an individual patient, the type and sequence of chemotherapy agents are often based on prior chemotherapy treatment history (i.e., agents used and time lapse from last chemotherapy), previous or persisting

Table 8.1 Commonly used single agent chemotherapy in metastatic triple-negative breast cancer

Drug	Dose	Frequency
Docetaxel	75–100 mg/m²	Day 1 of 21 day cycle
Paclitaxel	80 mg/m²	Weekly
Nab-paclitaxel	100–150 mg/m²	Days 1, 8, and 15 of 28 day cycle
Doxorubicin	60 mg/m²	Day 1 of 21 day cycle
Epirubicin	60 mg/m²	Day 1 of 21 day cycle
	90 mg/m²	Day 1 of 21 day cycle
Pegylated liposomal doxorubicin	40–50 mg/m²	Day 1 of 28 day cycle
Cisplatin	60–75 mg/m²	Day 1 of 21 day cycle
Carboplatin	AUC 6	Day 1 of 21–28 day cycle
	AUC 2	Days 1, 8, and 15 of 21 day cycle
Capecitabine[a]	1000–1250 mg/m²	Twice a day, days 1–14 of 21 day cycle
Gemcitabine	800–1250 mg/m²	Days 1, 8, and 15 of 28 day cycle
Vinorelbine	20–30 mg/m²	Days 1, 8, and 15 of 21 day cycle
Eribulin	1.4 mg/m²	Days 1 and 8 of 21 day cycle
Ixabepilone	40 mg/m²	Day 1 of 21 day cycle
Cyclophosphamide	600 mg/m²	Day 1 of 21 day cycle

Abbreviation: *AUC*, area under the curve
[a]Orally administered

toxicities from prior chemotherapy, and patient preference. Treatment with chemotherapy for metastatic TNBC is typically continued until disease progression or significant toxicity. With regards to the concept of maintenance or continual treatment, a 2011 meta-analysis analyzed 11 trials of 2300 treatment-naive patients with metastatic breast cancer, some of whom were triple-negative. A meta-analysis demonstrated that compared to intermittent treatment, continuous chemotherapy was associated with improved progression-free survival (PFS) and overall survival (OS) in metastatic breast cancer [24]. A randomized trial further evaluated the role of duration of chemotherapy in metastatic breast cancer. In this study, 324 patients with metastatic breast cancer (25% of whom were triple-negative) who achieved at least stable disease on paclitaxel and gemcitabine (PG) were randomized to observation or maintenance PG chemotherapy until disease progression. Maintenance chemotherapy resulted in better 6-month PFS rate (60% vs. 36%) and OS (32 vs. 24 months) at the cost of higher incidence of adverse events [25]. In a post hoc subset analysis, the improved outcomes with maintenance chemotherapy were primarily noted among young patients (<50 years of age) and patients with ER/PR-negative disease who had previously responded to chemotherapy and had predominantly visceral disease. Based on these observations, it is generally recommended that metastatic TNBC patients who are responding to chemotherapy continue beyond best response, especially if treatment-associated toxicities are tolerable and limited.

We briefly discuss the various chemotherapy classes commonly utilized in the treatment of metastatic TNBC. Given the lack of desirable outcomes with clinically available chemotherapy for metastatic TNBC, we encourage patient participation in clinical trials when available and feasible. At present, there are no clinically available predictive markers to aid in selection of specific chemotherapy agents in the treatment of metastatic TNBC, with the exception of germline *BRCA* status for platinum-based drugs (discussed below).

8.4   Taxanes

Taxanes are typically employed as first-line treatment for most patients with metastatic TNBC, especially if time lapse between neoadjuvant or adjuvant taxane exposure and development of metastatic disease is >12 months. Taxanes are among the most active agents for breast cancer. Docetaxel, paclitaxel, and nab-paclitaxel are often effective in the metastatic TNBC setting. When comparing the taxanes, the choice can be based on the safety and toxicity profile as well as on patient preference for scheduling. For docetaxel, every 3-week dosing is preferred as in the adjuvant setting. Every 3-week dosing was demonstrated to be superior compared to the weekly schedule [26]. Doses of docetaxel administered in the metastatic setting range from 80 to 100 mg/m^2 every 3 weeks. Every 3-week docetaxel is more myelosuppressive when compared with other taxanes given weekly; however, the risk of neuropathy is less with this agent.

Paclitaxel can be administered weekly or every 3 weeks. However, weekly dosing is recommended for breast cancer, as a meta-analysis has demonstrated superior efficacy of the weekly schedule compared to an every 3-week schedule in the metastatic setting and in the adjuvant setting as well [27]. The preferred dosing and scheduling of paclitaxel is 80–100 mg/m^2 on days 1, 8, and 15 of a 28-day cycle [26]. An important toxicity of paclitaxel is the potential for allergic reactions as a result of the required Cremophor solution. Thus, this agent requires steroid pre-medication with at least the first three to four doses. Paclitaxel can safely be administered with mild to moderate hepatic dysfunction with dose modifications, unlike docetaxel, which should be avoided in this setting.

Nab-paclitaxel has been demonstrated to have activity similar to paclitaxel in metastatic breast cancer [28–30]. Due to the lower risk of infusion reactions compared with either paclitaxel or docetaxel, nab-paclitaxel does not require steroid premedication, which may be appealing for patients who are at risk for significant hyperglycemia or who cannot tolerate systemic steroids.

8.5   Anthracyclines

Anthracyclines form the backbone of neoadjuvant and adjuvant chemotherapy for TNBC, which makes their application in the metastatic setting somewhat limited, especially given cumulative risk for cardiotoxicity. However, for patients who either did not receive these agents in the early stage setting or present with de novo metastatic TNBC, anthracyclines have a definite role. Doxorubicin, epirubicin, and pegylated liposomal doxorubicin are the three anthracycline agents available for treatment of metastatic breast cancer. Doxorubicin and epirubicin have not been compared head to head in metastatic breast cancer, and the choice between the two is typically based on institutional preferences and cost. In unselected metastatic breast cancer, pegylated liposomal doxorubicin administered every 4 weeks appeared to be equally active and less toxic compared to doxorubicin administered every 3 weeks [31]. The activity of pegylated liposomal doxorubicin monotherapy in metastatic TNBC is not well known. The risk for cumulative cardiac toxicity limits the duration of anthracycline-based therapy in the metastatic setting. Agents like dexrazoxane may minimize the risk of anthracycline-related cardiac toxicity when prolonged treatment is indicated. However, this scenario is not very frequent for metastatic TNBC given the short durations of responses to most chemotherapeutic agents.

8.6   Platinum Agents

Sporadic and germline *BRCA* mutation-associated TNBC share several pathological and molecular similarities [30–32]. The phenotypic and molecular similarities between *BRCA1* mutation-associated and sporadic TNBC has suggested that a significant proportion of *BRCA* wild-type TNBCs may involve the *BRCA1* pathway dysfunction through alternative mechanisms. Thus, *BRCA1*-directed therapeutic approaches, such as platinum agents, are being explored for the general population of TNBC. Platinum agents are not new to the treatment of breast cancer. In the 1980s, cisplatin was evaluated in advanced breast cancer in two phase II studies and demonstrated significant single-agent frontline activity, with response rates in the range of 50–54% [33, 34]. Due to its toxicity, cisplatin was subsequently abandoned and replaced by other active agents with more favorable toxicity profiles, such as taxanes and fluoropyrimidines. More recently, there has been renewed interest in exploring platinum agents in TNBC and *BRCA* mutation-associated breast cancers.

Repair of platinum-induced interstrand crosslinks invokes *BRCA1*-mediated homologous recombination (HR), and there is abundant clinical and in vitro evidence that *BRCA1*-deficient cells are hypersensitive to platinum agents [35–37]. Observational studies and small neoadjuvant and metastatic studies have demonstrated that *BRCA*-mutation-associated breast cancers are very sensitive to platinum agents [36–41]. In a phase II study, single-agent cisplatin yielded an impressive 80% response rate in *BRCA1* mutation-associated metastatic breast cancer [37]. A non-randomized study (TBCRC009) also demonstrated that response rate to platinum in first- or second-line treatment of metastatic TNBC was significantly higher in germline *BRCA* mutation carriers versus noncarriers (54% vs. 19%) [42].

The recent randomized phase III Triple-negative Breast Cancer Trial (TNT) compared first-line treatment carboplatin vs. docetaxel in unselected metastatic TNBC [41]. TNT randomized 376 patients with metastatic TNBC to either carboplatin (AUC 6 every 21 days) or docetaxel (100 mg/m² every 21 days). Carboplatin and docetaxel were equal in efficacy in unselected patients. However, in patients with *BRCA1/2* germline mutation, carboplatin yielded a superior response rate and PFS compared to docetaxel. Patients with germline *BRCA1/2* mutation were noted to have a doubling of response with carboplatin compared to docetaxel (68% vs. 33%) and demonstrated a median PFS of 6.8 months with carboplatin compared to 4.8 months with docetaxel. In summary, TNT demonstrated that single-agent platinum chemotherapy is superior to taxane in patients with germline *BRCA* mutation, highlighting the importance of germline *BRCA* status in informing therapy decisions for patients with metastatic TNBC. Besides germline *BRCA* status, no other biomarker-selected group could be identified that derived preferential benefit from platinum over taxane in the metastatic setting [43]. Given the molecular heterogeneity of TNBC, it is very likely that platinum agents will benefit only a subgroup of patients with TNBC. Ongoing and future translational studies (described in the below section) are focusing on identifying TNBC patients most likely to benefit from platinum therapy.

8.7   Antimetabolites

8.7.1   Capecitabine

The efficacy of capecitabine monotherapy has not been prospectively studied in metastatic TNBC. Some observations can be made regarding its efficacy from subgroup analyses of prospective trials. In the metastatic setting, two randomized phase III trials compared capecitabine plus ixabepilone to capecitabine monotherapy in 1712 patients treated with prior anthracycline and taxane therapy. In a combined subgroup analysis, 857 patients received capecitabine alone, of whom 208 patients had TNBC. The overall response rate (ORR) and median PFS in the capecitabine monotherapy arm were 25% and 4.2 months, respectively, in the overall population but only 15% and 1.7 months in the TNBC subgroup [32]. A single-arm phase II study of capecitabine with bevacizumab reported better efficacy of this combination in the ER-positive subgroup compared to TNBC. The overall response rate was 47% for ER-positive patients compared to 27% for TNBC, with time to progression 8.9 months for ER-positive patients compared to 4.0 months for TNBC [33]. These observations suggest that in patients previously treated with taxane and anthracycline, capecitabine monotherapy displays very modest activity. Additional data are needed before concluding that capecitabine has limited activity in TNBC. This agent continues to be one of the choices available to clinicians for treatment of metastatic TNBC, especially in the second line setting and beyond.

8.7.2   Gemcitabine

Gemcitabine (a pyrimidine antimetabolite) monotherapy demonstrates some activity in pretreated metastatic TNBC, with ORR ranging from 16% to 37% [34–36]. Gemcitabine is one of the available treatment options in the setting of anthracycline, taxane, and platinum failure, although its efficacy as a single agent specifically in metastatic TNBC is not well studied. Gemcitabine has been studied in combination with other chemotherapy agents, including taxane or platinum compounds, in metastatic TNBC, and these regimens are discussed in the section on combination chemotherapy.

8.8   Drugs that Target Microtubules

8.8.1   Vinorelbine

Vinorelbine, a semisynthetic vinca alkaloid, is another commonly used metastatic breast cancer chemotherapy agent and demonstrates modest single-agent activity in heavily pretreated patients (ORR: 25–45%) [37–39]. This agent has also not been studied specifically in the metastatic TNBC population.

8.8.2   Eribulin Mesylate

Eribulin mesylate is a non-taxane inhibitor of microtubule dynamics of the halichondrin class of antineoplastic drugs [40, 41]. A synthetic analogue of halichondrin B, eribulin was isolated from the marine sponge *Halichondria okadai*. It is designed to inhibit microtubule polymerization, resulting in apoptosis through an irreversible mitotic block at the G2-M phases [42]. Activity of eribulin in metastatic breast cancer was demonstrated in a phase III trial (EMBRACE) of 762 heavily pretreated patients who were randomly assigned to eribulin or treatment of physician's choice [43]. Treatment with eribulin significantly improved OS (median, 13.1 vs. 10.6 months). A subsequent randomized trial failed to demonstrate superiority of eribulin over capecitabine as first-, second-, or third-line therapy in metastatic breast cancer patients previously treated with anthracycline and taxane [44]. Data from these two phase III trials of eribulin were pooled to assess whether specific patient subgroups previously treated with an anthracycline and a taxane benefited from eribulin [45]. Subgroup analysis demonstrated that patients with HER2-negative and TNBC benefitted from eribulin. Patients with metastatic TNBC demonstrated an OS of 12.9 months with eribulin treatment, compared with 8.2 months with standard chemotherapy drugs (HR = 0.74, P = 0.0006). Eribulin represents a valuable addition to the chemotherapy armamentarium for the treatment of metastatic TNBC.

8.8.3 Epothilones

Epothilones can cause cell cycle arrest and apoptosis, and also work by stabilizing microtubules through the binding of the paclitaxel binding site [46]. The epothilones, however, bind to the microtubule in a manner different from the taxanes and are structurally different [47]. As such, these compounds have demonstrated potential for treatment of taxane-resistant tumors, including those that are refractory to multiple classes of agents.

Two randomized phase III trials (BMS 046 and BMS 048) evaluated the efficacy and safety of ixabepilone/capecitabine combination versus capecitabine alone. In BMS 046 and BMS 048, patients with metastatic disease who had been pretreated with or were resistant to an anthracycline and a taxane were included [15, 48, 49]. In both of these trials, improved PFS and ORR were noted with addition of ixabepilone to capecitabine.

In a preplanned pooled analysis from both trials, for 443 patients with metastatic TNBC, the addition of ixabepilone to capecitabine improved ORR (31% vs. 15%) and median PFS (4.2 vs. 1.7 months) over that seen with single-agent capecitabine [50]. Ixabepilone monotherapy was evaluated in a single-arm trial of 126 patients with metastatic or locally advanced breast cancer who had previously received an anthracycline, a taxane, and capecitabine and who had disease progression or received a minimum required cumulative dose. Single-agent ORR in this heavily pretreated setting was 12.4%. Ixabepilone was approved by the United States Food and Drug Administration (FDA) in 2007 as monotherapy for the treatment of metastatic breast cancer patients whose tumors were resistant/refractory to anthracyclines, taxanes, and capecitabine, or in combination with capecitabine in the setting of resistance/contraindication to anthracycline and taxane. Given its approval in such later line therapy, usefulness of this drug in clinic is often limited by its toxicities, including neuropathy, hematologic toxicities, and fatigue.

Alternate dosing schedules of ixabepilone have also been investigated in single-arm studies and appear to be associated with less toxicity [51, 52]. However, larger studies that could support routine clinical use of such alternate dose schedules have not been undertaken.

8.9   Combination Chemotherapy

While monotherapy with single-agent chemotherapy is preferred in most cases of metastatic TNBC, a chemotherapy doublet may be desired in situations of rapidly progressive disease and impending visceral crisis. Combination chemotherapy regimens have been explored generally in metastatic breast cancer with few studies that have focused specifically on the TNBC subtype [53–57]. Most doublet regimens tested have employed either a taxane or platinum as one of the chemotherapeutic agents. Several small phase I and II clinical trials of doublet chemotherapy regimens in first- and second-line metastatic setting have yielded ORR ranging from 20% to 85% [53, 56, 58–61]. In anthracycline-pretreated patients with metastatic breast cancer, unselected for breast cancer subtype, capecitabine plus docetaxel was superior to single-agent docetaxel therapy, yielding an ORR of 42% and median PFS of 6.1 months [62]. A small phase II study demonstrated an ORR of 85% and median PFS of 9.2 months with first-line combination treatment of nab-paclitaxel plus weekly carboplatin and bevacizumab [60]. The carboplatin plus gemcitabine combination has demonstrated an ORR of 32–34% and median PFS of 5.5–6.5 months in first-line setting (about two-thirds of patients in these trials received prior neo/adjuvant taxane) [55, 56]. In the setting of previous taxane treatment for metastatic disease or relapse within 2 years of neoadjuvant or adjuvant taxane, the carboplatin plus gemcitabine regimen yields an ORR of 25% and median PFS of 4.4 months [55]. Recently a randomized phase II trial (tnAcity) compared three chemotherapy doublets (nab-paclitaxel/gemcitabine, nab-paclitaxel/carboplatin, carboplatin/gemcitabine) in first-line treatment of metastatic TNBC [57]. This randomized phase II trial demonstrated superior ORR in the nab-paclitaxel/carboplatin arm (72%) compared to nab-paclitaxel/gemcitabine (39%) or gemcitabine/carboplatin (44%). Similar to ORR results, PFS was also significantly longer with nab-paclitaxel/carboplatin vs. either nab-paclitaxel/gemcitabine (median PFS, 7.4 vs. 5.4 months, $P = 0.03$) or gemcitabine/carboplatin (median PFS 7.4 vs. 6.0 months, $P = 0.02$) [57]. Over 60% of patients in tnAcity had received prior neoadjuvant or adjuvant taxane and two-thirds had received prior neoadjuvant or adjuvant anthracycline. Results from tnAcity demonstrate robust activity of taxane-platinum combination in first-line treatment of metastatic TNBC, especially when the time lapse is >12 months from neo/adjuvant taxane or when there has been no prior neo/adjuvant taxane exposure. In our opinion, a platinum/taxane combination should be the preferred combination in situations where a doublet is desired, such as rapidly progressive symptomatic disease.

8.10   PARP Inhibitors

Poly (ADP-ribose) polymerase (PARP) enzymes recognize DNA damage and facilitate DNA repair to maintain genomic stability. Preclinical studies demonstrate that PARP inhibition in the presence of *BRCA* deficiency leads to synthetic lethality [63–65]. PARP inhibitors have shown preclinical and clinical activity in targeting tumors with pre-existing DNA repair defects, in particular *BRCA1*- and *BRCA2*-deficient advanced breast and ovarian cancers [64–71]. A PARP inhibitor olaparib has been approved as monotherapy by the FDA as a first-in-class drug to treat germline *BRCA* mutation-associated advanced refractory ovarian cancers. Several ongoing studies are assessing the activity of PARP inhibitors either alone or in combination with chemotherapy for germline *BRCA*-associated early and metastatic breast cancers. OlympiAD, was a randomized, open-label, phase III trial, that compared olaparib monotherapy to physician's choice chemotherapy (capecitabine, eribulin, or vinorelbine) in patients with HER2-negative metastatic breast cancer who had received <3 prior lines of chemotherapy for metastatic disease and carried a germline *BRCA* mutation [72]. This trial demonstrated a significant benefit of olaparib over non-platinum chemotherapy. Median PFS was significantly longer in the olaparib group than in the chemotherapy group (7.0 months vs. 4.2 months, $P < 0.001$). The response rate in the olaparib group was approximately double the rate in the chemotherapy group (59.9% vs. 28.8%). No significant difference in OS was observed between the two arms, but the trial was not powered to assess differences in OS. The median time to the onset of a response was similar with olaparib. Chemotherapy is an important consideration for patients with symptomatic or rapidly progressing disease. The trial was not powered to detect any differences in treatment effect by subgroup (i.e., hormone receptor positive vs. triple-negative, prior platinum use vs. not, *BRCA1* vs. *BRCA2* mutation). Since platinum agents were not included as treatment options in the control group, the trial cannot address the relative benefits of olaparib over platinum-based chemotherapy in patients with *BRCA* mutation- associated breast cancer. It is noteworthy that the response rate of 59.9% and the median PFS of 7.0 months observed in OlympiAD are similar to the response rate of 68.0% and median PFS of 6.8 months noted with first-line carboplatin in *BRCA* mutation carriers with TNBC in the TNT study [73]. In summary, OlympiAD is the first randomized trial to demonstrate superiority of a PARP inhibitor over non-platinum chemotherapy in patients with *BRCA* mutation-associated metastatic breast cancer. When comparing across different studies, various PARP inhibitors including veliparib, olaparib, rucaparib, and talazoparib have typically demonstrated ORR ranging from 26% to 40% as monotherapy in germline *BRCA* mutation-associated metastatic breast cancer [67, 69, 71, 74, 75]. Variability of response rates is likely due to heterogeneity of patient population based on extent of prior treatment and platinum exposure across trials. Results of a phase II study of talazoparib following platinum or multiple cytotoxic regimens in advanced breast cancer patients with germline *BRCA1/2* mutations (ABRAZO) were recently presented [76]. The ORR with talazoparib monotherapy was 21% in patients who had responded to prior platinum therapy and 37% in patients who had received three or more prior lines of chemotherapy but no platinum agent.

PARP inhibitors are an important class of therapeutic agents for *BRCA*-mutation associated metastatic breast cancer, specifically for the TNBC subgroup which otherwise has limited treatment options. Additional studies that investigate the differential treatment effects of PARP inhibitors among breast cancer subtypes based on hormone and HER2 status and efficacy of these agents in comparison to platinum agents or in the setting of prior platinum exposure will be needed for refinement of the treatment roadmap for patients with *BRCA* mutation-associated metastatic TNBC.

8.11   Chemotherapy in the Setting of Liver Dysfunction

Chemotherapy selection in the setting of liver dysfunction poses a challenge for physicians, as many chemotherapeutic agents undergo hepatic metabolism. Furthermore, since the liver is one of the common sites of involvement by breast cancer, often the liver dysfunction may be secondary to extensive liver metastasis. Unfortunately, most clinical trials typically exclude patients with impaired hepatic function, and much of what is known about individual chemotherapeutic agents in the setting of liver dysfunction is based on small, retrospective studies. Capecitabine, cyclophosphamide, carboplatin, and cisplatin can typically be used without dose adjustments in setting of mild to moderate liver dysfunction. Taxanes, anthracyclines, vinorelbine, and gemcitabine typically require dose reductions in presence of mild to moderate liver dysfunction, with the exception of nab-paclitaxel, which does not require dose reductions in setting of mild impairment. We recommend close monitoring for chemotherapy-specific side effects when treating patients with hepatic dysfunction with chemotherapy.

8.12   Systemic Treatment in the Setting of Isolated
         Local or Regional Recurrence

Patients with ipsilateral local and regional recurrences (ILRR) have a high risk of developing distant metastases and dying from breast cancer. Five-year survival probabilities have been reported between 45% and 80% after isolated locoregional recurrence [77]. There is a paucity of data to inform recommendations on systemic treatment in patients who can undergo successful locoregional treatment and have no other evidence of systemic disease. The International Breast Cancer Study Group (IBCSG) conducted the Chemotherapy as Adjuvant for Locally Recurrent breast cancer (CALOR) trial in collaboration with the Breast International Group (BIG) and NSABP (IBCSG 27-02, BIG 1-02, NSABP B-37) to establish whether chemotherapy improves the outcome of patients with ILRR who undergo surgical resection of locally recurrent breast cancer [78]. The CALOR trial randomized 162 patients who underwent surgical resection of locally recurrent breast cancer to post-excision chemotherapy treatment (of physician's choice) or to no chemotherapy. Chemotherapy was found to reduce both distant and second local failures. Five-year disease-free survival was 69% in the chemotherapy group compared to 57% in the control group. This effect of chemotherapy was more notable in the ER-negative group, reducing the relative risk of relapse by about two-thirds (5-year DFS 67 versus 35%, HR 0.32) and reducing risk of death by almost 60% (5-year OS 79 vs. 69%, HR 0.43). These findings provide evidence that isolated breast cancer recurrences are probably a marker of concurrent occult systemic disease and that a second adjuvant course of chemotherapy should be recommended in this population of patients, specifically in patients with triple-negative disease.

8.13   Systemic Treatment in the Setting of Brain Metastasis

Compared to patients with other breast cancer subtypes, patients with TNBC have an increased risk of brain metastasis as the site of initial recurrence. The 5-year cumulative incidence of brain metastasis as a first site of recurrence for patients with TNBC has been reported to be 3%, 5%, and 10% with stage I, II, and III disease, respectively [79]. One study found the incidence of brain metastases at or following the diagnosis of metastatic breast cancer to be 46% [80].

Retrospective analyses suggest that the prognosis of breast cancer patients with brain metastases as a whole is improving, and this appears to be primarily a result of advances in systemic therapy, which have led to better control of disease outside the central nervous system (CNS). However, the prognosis of patients with metastatic TNBC and CNS metastases remains poor. In one series of 53 patients, the median survival after CNS recurrence in metastatic TNBC population was found to be 4.9 months [80]. Other published series have reported median survival ranging from 2.9 to 4.0 months in patients with metastatic TNBC [81–84].

The approach to the treatment of patients with brain metastasis is standard, regardless of breast cancer type, with treatment options generally based on prognosis and level of control of systemic disease. Local therapeutic options include surgical resection, stereotactic radiosurgery, and whole brain radiation therapy. Treatment of intracranial disease with systemic agents is limited by the ability of drugs to achieve sufficient concentration in the CNS. Novel approaches that address this issue are clearly needed. A preclinical study of carboplatin and the PARP inhibitor veliparib in mouse models of TNBC with brain metastasis demonstrated that both agents reached CNS tumors, as evidenced by evaluation of dynamic changes in gene expression and intracranial tumor PARP levels [85]. This strategy is now being investigated in a randomized phase II SWOG 1416 trial which specifically includes a TNBC progressive brain metastases cohort. Patients in this trial will be randomized to cisplatin with or without veliparib. Another promising agent in this space is etirinotecan pegol, a long-acting topoisomerase inhibitor, which, compared with irinotecan, prolongs the elimination half-life of the active metabolite SN38 from 2 to 50 days. Etirinotecan pegol crosses the blood–tumor barrier, leading to preferential accumulation and retention in brain tumor, and animal studies have demonstrated efficacy of this agent in treatment of brain metastasis [86]. The open-label phase III BEACON trial compared etirinotecan pegol with physician's choice of single-agent chemotherapy in a pretreated population of patients with HER2-negative metastatic breast cancer. This study did not meet its primary endpoint of improvement in OS [87]. Planned subgroup analysis from the BEACON trial demonstrated that etirinotecan pegol significantly prolonged OS compared with single-agent chemotherapy in patients with a history of brain metastasis (10.0 months vs. 4.8 months, $P = 0.0099$). An ongoing phase III trial is comparing etirinotecan pegol to chemotherapy of physician's choice in patients with metastatic breast cancer who have stable brain metastases and have been previously treated with an anthracycline, a taxane, and capecitabine (NCT02915744).

8.14 Use of Bone Modifying Agents

Bone metastasis can cause significant morbidity for patients with metastatic breast cancer [88]. ASCO guidelines recommend incorporation of a bone modifying agent in the treatment of patients with bone metastases from solid tumors, including breast cancer. This recommendation is to continue such treatment until there has been a decline in the health status of the patient such that treatment is no longer thought to offer substantial benefit to the patient [89].

There are two classes of agents used commonly for osteoclast inhibition in patients with bone metastases from breast cancer: bisphosphonates (zoledronic acid) and receptor activator of nuclear factor kappa B ligand (RANKL) inhibitors (denosumab). Selection of one agent over another can be determined by patient preference regarding route of administration, tolerance, and cost. Both of these agents are typically dosed every 4 weeks. For zoledronic acid there are now data from OPTIMIZE-2 and ZOOM trials to support less frequent dosing of every 12 weeks for patients with metastatic breast cancer who have been on bisphosphonate therapy for 9–12 months [90]. If zoledronic acid is being used, we suggest starting out with every 4-week dosing, especially in setting of symptomatic and/or extensive osseous disease, and then after 9–12 months of therapy, extending the interval to every 12 weeks. Currently, there is limited data for less frequent dosing of denosumab, but ongoing trials are addressing this question.

8.15 Identification and Development of Novel Targeted Agents - Promise on the Horizon

In recent years, significant progress has been made in unraveling the biological diversity of TNBC and linking gene expression patterns to distinct molecular subtypes with potential therapeutic associations [91–94]. Using gene expression from publicly available data sets, Lehmann and colleagues classified TNBC initially into seven molecular subtypes, and recently refined the classification into four molecular subtypes: basal-like 1 (BL1), basal-like 2 (BL2), mesenchymal (M), and luminal androgen receptor-like (LAR) [92, 95]. Based on identification of cell lines corresponding to each subtype, they also demonstrated that each subtype may be responsive to different targeted therapies [92]. The methodology of the Lehmann et al. molecular classification has recently been simplified to a RNA-seq platform to better fit individual clinical samples [96]. Development and refinement of next-generation sequencing has improved our understanding of the prevalence of somatic mutations in various cancers. However, absence of high-frequency, targetable oncogenic drivers in TNBC has hindered the development of successful therapeutic strategies [18, 94]. In TNBC, TP53 mutation is reported to be the most frequent clonal event (53.8%), followed by PIK3CA mutations [94, 97]. To date there are no available effective agents to target TP53 mutations, although efforts to develop such agents are ongoing. The frequency and coexistence of various genomic alterations in TNBC also undergo evolution under the pressure of systemic chemotherapy. For example, profiling of residual TNBC tumor tissue after neoadjuvant chemotherapy revealed higher frequency of several potentially targetable alterations compared with paired basal-like primary breast cancers in The Cancer Genome Atlas. These included alterations in the PTEN/PI3K/mTOR pathway (noted in 40% of samples), and amplifications of JAK2, CDK6, CCND1, CCND2, and CCND3.

With these advances in our ability to understand the diversity of TNBC has come the potential to identify molecular subtypes that are candidates for various targeted treatment approaches. Many ongoing studies are evaluating targeted agents for use as single agents or in combination for TNBC (Table 8.2).

Table 8.2 Selected clinical trials of novel agents in metastatic triple-negative breast cancer

Class	Trial details	Phase	NCT number
Immune checkpoint inhibitors			
	Nab-paclitaxel ± atezolizumab (MPDL3280A) in previously untreated TNBC (IMpassion130)	III	NCT02425891
	Pembrolizumab plus doxorubicin in metastatic TNBC	II	NCT02648477
	Nivolumab in combination with various chemotherapy drugs in advanced TNBC (TONIC trial)	II	NCT02499367
	Phase I/II study of PDR001 in patients with advanced malignancies	I/II	NCT02404441
	Study of single-agent pembrolizumab versus single-agent chemotherapy for metastatic TNBC (MK-3475-119/KEYNOTE-119)	III	NCT02555657
	Study of safety and efficacy of durvalumab in combination with paclitaxel in metastatic TNBC patients	I/II	NCT02628132
	Phase I/II study of cisplatin plus romidepsin and nivolumab in metastatic TNBC or *BRCA* mutation-associated locally recurrent or metastatic breast cancer	I/II	NCT02393794
	A study of avelumab in combination with other cancer immunotherapies in advanced malignancies (JAVELIN Medley)	II	NCT02554812
	Randomized phase II study of atezolizumab and entinostat in patients with advanced TNBC (Phase 1b lead in)	I/II	NCT02708680
	Pilot study of durvalumab and Vigil in advanced women's cancers	II	NCT02725489
Poly(ADP-ribose) polymerase (PARP) inhibitors			
	Carboplatin and paclitaxel with or without veliparib (ABT-888) in patients with *BRCA* mutation-associated advanced breast cancer	II	NCT01506609
	Talazoparib (BMN 673) monotherapy versus physician's choice chemotherapy in metastatic breast cancer patients with germline *BRCA1/2* mutations (EMBRACA study)	III	NCT01945775

Table 8.2 (continued)

Class	Trial details	Phase	NCT number
	Cisplatin ± ABT-888 (veliparib) in *BRCA*-associated HER2-negative metastatic breast cancer and BRCAness phenotype metastatic TNBC (SWOG 1416)	II	NCT02595905
	Talazoparib (BMN 673) monotherapy in *BRCA1/2* wild-type advanced TNBC with homologous recombination deficiency as assessed by the HRD assay (Myriad), or germline/somatic mutation in homologous recombination pathway genes	II	NCT02401347
Androgen-targeted therapy			
	Bicalutamide for the treatment of AR-positive, estrogen receptor-negative, progesterone receptor-negative metastatic breast cancer	II	NCT00468715
	Bicalutamide in treating patients with AR-positive metastatic TNBC	II	NCT02353988
	Transdermal CR1447 (4-OH-testosterone) in endocrine-responsive/HER2-negative and triple-negative/AR-positive metastatic or locally advanced breast cancer	II	NCT02067741
	Bicalutamide versus chemotherapy in first-line treatment of AR-positive metastatic TNBC	III	NCT03055312
	Ribociclib (LEE011), a CDK 4/6 inhibitor, in combination with bicalutamide in advanced AR-positive TNBC (BRE15–024)	I/II	NCT03090165
	Enzalutamide in patients with advanced, AR-positive TNBC	II	NCT01889238
	Pembrolizumab and enobosarm in treating patients with AR-positive metastatic TNBC	II	NCT02971761
PI3K-AKT-mTOR pathway inhibitors			
	Paclitaxel with or without AZD5363 in first-line metastatic TNBC (PAKT)	II	NCT02423603
	BYL719 monotherapy in advanced metastatic breast cancer (second-line setting)	II	NCT02506556
	BYL719 with nab-paclitaxel in HER2-negative metastatic breast cancer	I/II	NCT02379247
	BKM120 in combination with the PARP inhibitor olaparib in metastatic TNBC	I	NCT01623349
Antibody-drug conjugate			
	Glembatumumab vedotin (CDX-011) versus capecitabine in patients with metastatic, gpNMB overexpressing TNBC (METRIC)	II	NCT01997333
	Randomized, phase III trial of sacituzumab govitecan (IMMU-132) versus treatment of physician's choice in patients with mTNBC who received at least two prior treatments	III	NCT02574455
	Mirvetuximab soravtansine and gemcitabine in patients with FRa-positive recurrent ovarian, primary peritoneal, fallopian tube, endometrial, or triple-negative breast cancer	I	NCT02996825

(continued)

Table 8.2 (continued)

Class	Trial details	Phase	NCT number
Heat shock protein 90 (HSP90) and histone deacetylase (HDAC) inhibitors			
	AT13387 (HSP90 inhibitor) plus paclitaxel in advanced TNBC	I	NCT02474173
	Entinostat (HDAC inhibitor) plus azacitidine in advanced breast cancer	II	NCT01349959
Aurora kinase inhibitor	ENMD-2076 (Aurora + angiogenic kinase inhibitor) in previously treated locally advanced/metastatic TNBC	II	NCT01639248
Death receptors	Nab-paclitaxel with or without tigatuzumab in metastatic triple-negative breast cancer	II	NCT01307891
CSF1 inhibitor	PLX3397 and eribulin in patients with metastatic breast cancer, with phase II limited to TNBC	lb/II	NCT01596751

Abbreviations: *AR* androgen receptor, *CDK* cyclin-dependent kinase, *CSF*-1 colony stimulating factor 1, *FRa* folate receptor alpha, *gpNMB* transmembrane glycoprotein NMB, *HRD* homologous recombination deficiency, *mTOR* mechanistic target of rapamycin, *PI3K* phosphatidylinositol-3-kinase, *TNBC* triple-negative breast cancer

Conclusion

TNBC is a heterogeneous breast cancer subtype. The genetic and molecular heterogeneity of these tumors, shorter median time from relapse to death, and lack of currently identified treatment targets make the management of metastatic TNBC challenging. Due to the lack of FDA-approved targeted therapy, chemotherapy remains the mainstay of treatment for advanced disease. Sequential use of single-agent chemotherapy is the most widely practiced treatment strategy for metastatic TNBC, with the usual approach of treating until disease progression or intolerable toxicity. Commonly used chemotherapy agents include taxanes, anthracyclines, platinum salts, antimetabolites, vinca alkaloids, and non-taxane tubulin- polymerizing agents such as ixabepilone and eribulin. Several promising drug classes such as immune checkpoint inhibitors, antibody drug conjugates, PARP inhibitors, androgen receptor antagonists, and PI3K/AKT inhibitors are being investigated in clinical trials. Future research efforts should focus on studying targeted agents in biologically and molecularly identified subgroups of TNBC. It is through this process that meaningful strides will be made to improve the outcomes of patients with triple-negative metastatic disease.

References

1. Bauer KR, Brown M, Cress RD, Parise CA, Caggiano V. Descriptive analysis of estrogen receptor (ER)-negative, progesterone receptor (PR)-negative, and HER2-negative invasive breast cancer, the so-called triple-negative phenotype: a population-based study from the California Cancer Registry. Cancer. 2007;109(9):1721–8.
2. Hammond ME, Hayes DF, Wolff AC, Mangu PB, Temin S. American Society of Clinical Oncology/College of American Pathologists guideline recommendations for immunohistochemical testing of estrogen and progesterone receptors in breast cancer. J Oncol Pract. 2010;6(4):195–7.

3. Wolff AC, Hammond MEH, Hicks DG, Dowsett M, McShane LM, Allison KH, et al. Recommendations for human epidermal growth factor receptor 2 testing in breast cancer: American Society of Clinical Oncology/College of American Pathologists clinical practice guideline update. J Clin Oncol. 2013;31(31):3997–4013.
4. Kohler BA, Sherman RL, Howlader N, Jemal A, Ryerson AB, Henry KA, et al. Annual report to the nation on the status of cancer, 1975–2011, featuring incidence of breast cancer subtypes by race/ethnicity, poverty, and state. J Natl Cancer Inst. 2015;107(6):djv048.
5. Carey LA, Dees EC, Sawyer L, Gatti L, Moore DT, Collichio F, et al. The triple negative paradox: primary tumor chemosensitivity of breast cancer subtypes. Clin Cancer Res. 2007;13(8):2329–34.
6. Dent R, Trudeau M, Pritchard KI, Hanna WM, Kahn HK, Sawka CA, et al. Triple-negative breast cancer: clinical features and patterns of recurrence. Clin Cancer Res. 2007;13(15 Pt 1):4429–34.
7. Liedtke C, Mazouni C, Hess KR, Andre F, Tordai A, Mejia JA, et al. Response to neoadjuvant therapy and long-term survival in patients with triple-negative breast cancer. J Clin Oncol. 2008;26(8):1275–81.
8. Carlson RW, Allred DC, Anderson BO, Burstein HJ, Edge SB, Farrar WB, et al. Metastatic breast cancer, version 1.2012: featured updates to the NCCN guidelines. J Natl Compr Cancer Netw. 2012;10(7):821–9.
9. de Duenas EM, Hernandez AL, Zotano AG, Carrion RM, Lopez-Muniz JI, Novoa SA, et al. Prospective evaluation of the conversion rate in the receptor status between primary breast cancer and metastasis: results from the GEICAM 2009-03 ConvertHER study. Breast Cancer Res Treat. 2014;143(3):507–15.
10. Bussolati G, Leonardo E. Technical pitfalls potentially affecting diagnoses in immunohisto-chemistry. J Clin Pathol. 2008;61(11):1184–92.
11. Gruchy JR, Barnes PJ, Dakin Hache KA. CytoLyt(R) fixation and decalcification pretreatments alter antigenicity in normal tissues compared with standard formalin fixation. Appl Immunohistochem Mol Morphol. 2015;23(4):297–302.
12. Cheang MC, Voduc D, Bajdik C, Leung S, McKinney S, Chia SK, et al. Basal-like breast cancer defined by five biomarkers has superior prognostic value than triple-negative phenotype. Clin Cancer Res. 2008;14(5):1368–76.
13. Dent R, Hanna WM, Trudeau M, Rawlinson E, Sun P, Narod SA. Pattern of metastatic spread in triple-negative breast cancer. Breast Cancer Res Treat. 2009;115(2):423–8.
14. Swain SM, Baselga J, Kim SB, Ro J, Semiglazov V, Campone M, et al. Pertuzumab, trastuzumab, and docetaxel in HER2-positive metastatic breast cancer. N Engl J Med. 2015;372(8):724–34.
15. Thomas ES, Gomez HL, Li RK, Chung HC, Fein LE, Chan VF, et al. Ixabepilone plus capecitabine for metastatic breast cancer progressing after anthracycline and taxane treatment. J Clin Oncol. 2007;25(33):5210–7.
16. Bunnell C, Vahdat L, Schwartzberg L, Gralow J, Klimovsky J, Poulart V, et al. Phase I/II study of ixabepilone plus capecitabine in anthracycline-pretreated/resistant and taxane-resistant metastatic breast cancer. Clin Breast Cancer. 2008;8(3):234–41.
17. Gonzalez-Angulo AM, Timms KM, Liu S, Chen H, Litton JK, Potter J, et al. Incidence and outcome of BRCA mutations in unselected patients with triple receptor-negative breast cancer. Clin Cancer Res. 2011;17(5):1082–9.
18. Hartman AR, Kaldate RR, Sailer LM, Painter L, Grier CE, Endsley RR, et al. Prevalence of BRCA mutations in an unselected population of triple-negative breast cancer. Cancer. 2012;118(11):2787–95.
19. Sharma P, Klemp JR, Kimler BF, Mahnken JD, Geier LJ, Khan QJ, et al. Germline BRCA mutation evaluation in a prospective triple-negative breast cancer registry: implications for hereditary breast and/or ovarian cancer syndrome testing. Breast Cancer Res Treat. 2014;145(3):707–14.
20. Couch FJ, Hart SN, Sharma P, Toland AE, Wang X, Miron P, et al. Inherited mutations in 17 breast cancer susceptibility genes among a large triple-negative breast cancer cohort unselected for family history of breast cancer. J Clin Oncol. 2015;33(4):304–11.

21. Fossati R, Confalonieri C, Torri V, Ghislandi E, Penna A, Pistotti V, et al. Cytotoxic and hormonal treatment for metastatic breast cancer: a systematic review of published randomized trials involving 31,510 women. J Clin Oncol. 1998;16(10):3439–60.
22. Dear RF, McGeechan K, Jenkins MC, Barratt A, Tattersall MH, Wilcken N. Combination versus sequential single agent chemotherapy for metastatic breast cancer. Cochrane Database Syst Rev. 2013;12:CD008792.
23. Carrick S, Parker S, Thornton CE, Ghersi D, Simes J, Wilcken N. Single agent versus combination chemotherapy for metastatic breast cancer. Cochrane Database Syst Rev. 2009(2):Cd003372.
24. Gennari A, Stockler M, Puntoni M, Sormani M, Nanni O, Amadori D, et al. Duration of chemotherapy for metastatic breast cancer: a systematic review and meta-analysis of randomized clinical trials. J Clin Oncol. 2011;29(16):2144–9.
25. Park YH, Jung KH, Im SA, Sohn JH, Ro J, Ahn JH, et al. Phase III, multicenter, randomized trial of maintenance chemotherapy versus observation in patients with metastatic breast cancer after achieving disease control with six cycles of gemcitabine plus paclitaxel as first-line chemotherapy: KCSG-BR07-02. J Clin Oncol. 2013;31(14):1732–9.
26. Sparano JA, Wang M, Martino S, Jones V, Perez EA, Saphner T, et al. Weekly paclitaxel in the adjuvant treatment of breast cancer. N Engl J Med. 2008;358(16):1663–71.
27. Mauri D, Kamposioras K, Tsali L, Bristianou M, Valachis A, Karathanasi I, et al. Overall survival benefit for weekly vs. three-weekly taxanes regimens in advanced breast cancer: a meta-analysis. Cancer Treat Rev. 2010;36(1):69–74.
28. Ibrahim NK, Samuels B, Page R, Doval D, Patel KM, Rao SC, et al. Multicenter phase II trial of ABI-007, an albumin-bound paclitaxel, in women with metastatic breast cancer. J Clin Oncol. 2005;23(25):6019–26.
29. Gradishar WJ, Krasnojon D, Cheporov S, Makhson AN, Manikhas GM, Clawson A, et al. Significantly longer progression-free survival with nab-paclitaxel compared with docetaxel as first-line therapy for metastatic breast cancer. J Cin Oncol. 2009;27(22):3611–9.
30. Rugo HS, Barry WT, Moreno-Aspitia A, Lyss AP, Cirrincione C, Leung E, et al. Randomized phase III trial of paclitaxel once per week compared with nanoparticle albumin-bound Nab-paclitaxel once per week or ixabepilone with bevacizumab as first-line chemotherapy for locally recurrent or metastatic breast cancer: CALGB 40502/NCCTG N063H (Alliance). J Clin Oncol. 2015;33(21):2361–9.
31. O'Brien ME, Wigler N, Inbar M, Rosso R, Grischke E, Santoro A, et al. Reduced cardiotoxicity and comparable efficacy in a phase III trial of pegylated liposomal doxorubicin HCl (CAELYX/Doxil) versus conventional doxorubicin for first-line treatment of metastatic breast cancer. Ann Oncol. 2004;15(3):440–9.
32. Rugo H, Roche H, Thomas E, Blackwell K, Chung H, Lerzo G, et al. Ixabepilone plus capecitabine vs capecitabine in patients with triple negative tumors: a pooled analysis of patients from two large phase III clinical studies. Cancer Res. 2009;69(2 Supplement):3057.
33. Sledge G, Miller K, Moisa C, Gradishar W. Safety and efficacy of capecitabine (C) plus bevacizumab (B) as first-line in metastatic breast cancer. J Clin Oncol. 2007;25(18_suppl):1013.
34. Rha SY, Moon YH, Jeung HC, Kim YT, Sohn JH, Yang WI, et al. Gemcitabine monotherapy as salvage chemotherapy in heavily pretreated metastatic breast cancer. Breast Cancer Res Treat. 2005;90(3):215–21.
35. Blackstein M, Vogel CL, Ambinder R, Cowan J, Iglesias J, Melemed A. Gemcitabine as first-line therapy in patients with metastatic breast cancer: a phase II trial. Oncology. 2002;62(1):2–8.
36. Feher O, Vodvarka P, Jassem J, Morack G, Advani SH, Khoo KS, et al. First-line gemcitabine versus epirubicin in postmenopausal women aged 60 or older with metastatic breast cancer: a multicenter, randomized, phase III study. Ann Oncol. 2005;16(6):899–908.
37. Vogel C, O'Rourke M, Winer E, Hochster H, Chang A, Adamkiewicz B, et al. Vinorelbine as first-line chemotherapy for advanced breast cancer in women 60 years of age or older. Ann Oncol. 1999;10(4):397–402.
38. Martin M, Ruiz A, Munoz M, Balil A, Garcia-Mata J, Calvo L, et al. Gemcitabine plus vinorelbine versus vinorelbine monotherapy in patients with metastatic breast cancer previously

treated with anthracyclines and taxanes: final results of the phase III Spanish Breast Cancer Research Group (GEICAM) trial. Lancet Oncol. 2007;8(3):219–25.

39. Jones S, Winer E, Vogel C, Laufman L, Hutchins L, O'Rourke M, et al. Randomized comparison of vinorelbine and melphalan in anthracycline-refractory advanced breast cancer. J Clin Oncol. 1995;13(10):2567–74.

40. Jordan MA, Kamath K, Manna T, Okouneva T, Miller HP, Davis C, et al. The primary antimitotic mechanism of action of the synthetic halichondrin E7389 is suppression of microtubule growth. Mol Cancer Ther. 2005;4(7):1086–95.

41. Towle MJ, Salvato KA, Budrow J, Wels BF, Kuznetsov G, Aalfs KK, et al. In vitro and in vivo anticancer activities of synthetic macrocyclic ketone analogues of halichondrin B. Cancer Res. 2001;61(3):1013–21.

42. Okouneva T, Azarenko O, Wilson L, Littlefield BA, Jordan MA. Inhibition of centromere dynamics by eribulin (E7389) during mitotic metaphase. Mol Cancer Ther. 2008;7(7):2003–11.

43. Cortes J, O'Shaughnessy J, Loesch D, Blum JL, Vahdat LT, Petrakova K, et al. Eribulin monotherapy versus treatment of physician's choice in patients with metastatic breast cancer (EMBRACE): a phase 3 open-label randomised study. Lancet (London, England). 2011;377(9769):914–23.

44. Kaufman PA, Awada A, Twelves C, Yelle L, Perez EA, Velikova G, et al. Phase III open-label randomized study of eribulin mesylate versus capecitabine in patients with locally advanced or metastatic breast cancer previously treated with an anthracycline and a taxane. J Clin Oncol. 2015;33(6):594–601.

45. Twelves C, Cortes J, Vahdat L, Olivo M, He Y, Kaufman PA, et al. Efficacy of eribulin in women with metastatic breast cancer: a pooled analysis of two phase 3 studies. Breast Cancer Res Treat. 2014;148(3):553–61.

46. Altmann K-H, Wartmann M, O'Reilly T. Epothilones and related structures – a new class of microtubule inhibitors with potent in vivo antitumor activity. Biochim Biophys Acta. 2000;1470(3):M79–91.

47. Giannakakou P, Gussio R, Nogales E, Downing KH, Zaharevitz D, Bollbuck B, et al. A common pharmacophore for epothilone and taxanes: molecular basis for drug resistance conferred by tubulin mutations in human cancer cells. Proc Natl Acad Sci. 2000;97(6):2904–9.

48. Hortobagyi GN, Gomez HL, Li RK, Chung HC, Fein LE, Chan VF, et al. Analysis of overall survival from a phase III study of ixabepilone plus capecitabine versus capecitabine in patients with MBC resistant to anthracyclines and taxanes. Breast Cancer Res Treat. 2010;122(2):409–18.

49. Sparano JA, Vrdoljak E, Rixe O, Xu B, Manikhas A, Medina C, et al. Randomized phase III trial of ixabepilone plus capecitabine versus capecitabine in patients with metastatic breast cancer previously treated with an anthracycline and a taxane. J Clin Oncol. 2010;28(20):3256–63.

50. Perez EA, Patel T, Moreno-Aspitia A. Efficacy of ixabepilone in ER/PR/HER2-negative (triple-negative) breast cancer. Breast Cancer Res Treat. 2010;121(2):261–71.

51. Denduluri N, Low JA, Lee JJ, Berman AW, Walshe JM, Vatas U, et al. Phase II trial of ixabepilone, an epothilone B analog, in patients with metastatic breast cancer previously untreated with taxanes. J Clin Oncol. 2007;25(23):3421–7.

52. Low JA, Wedam SB, Lee JJ, Berman AW, Brufsky A, Yang SX, et al. Phase II clinical trial of ixabepilone (BMS-247550), an epothilone B analog, in metastatic and locally advanced breast cancer. J Clin Oncol. 2005;23(12):2726–34.

53. Chew HK, Doroshow JH, Frankel P, Margolin KA, Somlo G, Lenz HJ, et al. Phase II studies of gemcitabine and cisplatin in heavily and minimally pretreated metastatic breast cancer. J Clin Oncol. 2009;27(13):2163–9.

54. Delord JP, Puozzo C, Lefresne F, Bugat R. Combination chemotherapy of vinorelbine and cisplatin: a phase I pharmacokinetic study in patients with metastatic solid tumors. Anticancer Res. 2009;29(2):553–60.

55. Loesch D, Asmar L, McIntyre K, Doane L, Monticelli M, Paul D, et al. Phase II trial of gemcitabine/carboplatin (plus trastuzumab in HER2-positive disease) in patients with metastatic breast cancer. Clin Breast Cancer. 2008;8(2):178–86.

56. Yardley DA, Burris HA, Simons L, Spigel DR, Greco EA, Barton JH, et al. A phase II trial of gemcitabine/carboplatin with or without trastuzumab in the first-line treatment of patients with metastatic breast cancer. Clin Breast Cancer. 2008;8(5):425–31.
57. Yardley D, Coleman R, Conte P, Cortes J, Brufsky A, Shtivelband M, et al. *nab*-paclitaxel + carboplatin or gemcitabine vs gemcitabine/carboplatin as first-line treatment for patients with triple-negative metastatic breast cancer: Results from the randomized phase 2 portion of the tnAcity trial [abstract]. Cancer Res. 2017;77(4 Suppl):P5-15-03.
58. Rodler ET, Kurland BF, Griffin M, Gralow JR, Porter P, Yeh RF, et al. Phase I study of veliparib (ABT-888) combined with cisplatin and vinorelbine in advanced triple-negative breast cancer and/or BRCA mutation-associated breast cancer. Clin Cancer Res. 2016;22(12):2855–64.
59. Lobo C, Lopes G, Baez O, Castrellon A, Ferrell A, Higgins C, et al. Final results of a phase II study of nab-paclitaxel, bevacizumab, and gemcitabine as first-line therapy for patients with HER2-negative metastatic breast cancer. Breast Cancer Res Treat. 2010;123(2):427–35.
60. Hamilton E, Kimmick G, Hopkins J, Marcom PK, Rocha G, Welch R, et al. Nab-paclitaxel/bevacizumab/carboplatin chemotherapy in first-line triple negative metastatic breast cancer. Clin Breast Cancer. 2013;13(6):416–20.
61. Roy V, LaPlant BR, Gross GG, Bane CL, Palmieri FM. Phase II trial of weekly nab (nanoparticle albumin-bound)-paclitaxel (nab-paclitaxel) (Abraxane) in combination with gemcitabine in patients with metastatic breast cancer (N0531). Ann Oncol. 2009;20(3):449–53.
62. O'Shaughnessy J, Miles D, Vukelja S, Moiseyenko V, Ayoub J-P, Cervantes G, et al. Superior survival with capecitabine plus docetaxel combination therapy in anthracycline-pretreated patients with advanced breast cancer: Phase III trial results. J Clin Oncol. 2002;20(12):2812–23.
63. McCabe N, Turner NC, Lord CJ, Kluzek K, Bialkowska A, Swift S, et al. Deficiency in the repair of DNA damage by homologous recombination and sensitivity to poly(ADP-ribose) polymerase inhibition. Cancer Res. 2006;66(16):8109–15.
64. Farmer H, McCabe N, Lord CJ, Tutt AN, Johnson DA, Richardson TB, et al. Targeting the DNA repair defect in BRCA mutant cells as a therapeutic strategy. Nature. 2005;434(7035):917–21.
65. Bryant HE, Schultz N, Thomas HD, Parker KM, Flower D, Lopez E, et al. Specific killing of BRCA2-deficient tumours with inhibitors of poly(ADP-ribose) polymerase. Nature. 2005;434(7035):913–7.
66. Fong PC, Boss DS, Yap TA, Tutt A, Wu P, Mergui-Roelvink M, et al. Inhibition of poly(ADP-ribose) polymerase in tumors from BRCA mutation carriers. N Engl J Med. 2009;361(2):123–34.
67. Audeh MW, Carmichael J, Penson RT, Friedlander M, Powell B, Bell-McGuinn KM, et al. Oral poly(ADP-ribose) polymerase inhibitor olaparib in patients with BRCA1 or BRCA2 mutations and recurrent ovarian cancer: a proof-of-concept trial. Lancet (London, England). 2010;376(9737):245–51.
68. Tutt A, Robson M, Garber JE, Domchek SM, Audeh MW, Weitzel JN, et al. Oral poly(ADP-ribose) polymerase inhibitor olaparib in patients with BRCA1 or BRCA2 mutations and advanced breast cancer: a proof-of-concept trial. Lancet (London, England). 2010;376(9737):235–44.
69. Mina LA, Ramanathan RK, Wainberg ZA, Byers LA, Chugh R, Sachdev JC, et al. BMN673 is a PARP inhibitor in clinical development for the treatment of breast cancer patients with deleterious germline BRCA1 and 2 mutations [abstract]. Cancer Res. 2013;73(24 Suppl):P2-09-02
70. Sandhu SK, Schelman WR, Wilding G, Moreno V, Baird RD, Miranda S, et al. The poly(ADP-ribose) polymerase inhibitor niraparib (MK4827) in BRCA mutation carriers and patients with sporadic cancer: a phase 1 dose-escalation trial. Lancet Oncol. 2013;14(9):882–92.
71. Kaufman B, Shapira-Frommer R, Schmutzler RK, Audeh MW, Friedlander M, Balmana J, et al. Olaparib monotherapy in patients with advanced cancer and a germline BRCA1/2 mutation. J Clin Oncol. 2015;33(3):244–50.
72. Robson M, Im SA, Senkus E, Xu B, Domchek SM, Masuda N, et al. Olaparib for metastatic breast cancer in patients with a germline BRCA mutation. N Engl J Med. 2017;377:523–33.
73. Tutt A, Cheang M, Kilburn L, Tovey H, Gillett C, Pinder S, et al. *BRCA1* methylation status, silencing and treatment effect in the TNT trial: A randomized phase III trial of carboplatin com-

pared with docetaxel for patients with metastatic or recurrent locally advanced triple negative or BRCA1/2 breast cancer (CRUK/07/012) [abstract]. Cancer Res. 2017;77(4 Suppl):S6-01.
74. Shen Y, Rehman FL, Feng Y, Boshuizen J, Bajrami I, Elliott R, et al. BMN 673, a novel and highly potent PARP1/2 inhibitor for the treatment of human cancers with DNA repair deficiency. Clin Cancer Res. 2013;19(18):5003–15.
75. Somlo G, Frankel PH, Luu TH, Ma C, Arun B, Garcia A, et al. Phase II trial of single agent PARP inhibitor ABT-888 (veliparib [vel]) followed by postprogression therapy of vel with carboplatin (carb) in patients (pts) with stage BRCA-associated metastatic breast cancer (MBC): California Cancer Consortium trial PHII-96. J Clin Oncol. 2014;32(15_suppl):1021.
76. Turner N, Telli ML, Rugo HS, Mailiez A, Ettl J, Grischke EM, et al., editors. Final results of a phase 2 study of talazoparib (TALA) following platinum or multiple cytotoxic regimens in advanced breast cancer patients (pts) with germline BRCA1/2 mutations (ABRAZO). ASCO Annual Meeting 2017; Chicago, IL.
77. Wapnir IL, Aebi S, Geyer CE, Zahrieh D, Gelber RD, Anderson SJ, et al. A randomized clinical trial of adjuvant chemotherapy for radically resected locoregional relapse of breast cancer: IBCSG 27-02, BIG 1-02, and NSABP B-37. Clin Breast Cancer. 2008;8(3):287–92.
78. Aebi S, Gelber S, Anderson SJ, Lang I, Robidoux A, Martin M, et al. Chemotherapy for isolated locoregional recurrence of breast cancer (CALOR): a randomised trial. Lancet Oncol. 2014;15(2):156–63.
79. Dawood S, Lei X, Litton JK, Buchholz TA, Hortobagyi GN, Gonzalez-Angulo AM. Incidence of brain metastases as a first site of recurrence among women with triple receptor-negative breast cancer. Cancer. 2012;118(19):4652–9.
80. Lin NU, Claus E, Sohl J, Razzak AR, Arnaout A, Winer EP. Sites of distant recurrence and clinical outcomes in patients with metastatic triple-negative breast cancer: high incidence of central nervous system metastases. Cancer. 2008;113(10):2638–45.
81. Dawood S, Broglio K, Esteva FJ, Yang W, Kau SW, Islam R, et al. Survival among women with triple receptor-negative breast cancer and brain metastases. Ann Oncol. 2009;20(4):621–7.
82. Eichler AF, Kuter I, Ryan P, Schapira L, Younger J, Henson JW. Survival in patients with brain metastases from breast cancer: the importance of HER-2 status. Cancer. 2008;112(11):2359–67.
83. Nam BH, Kim SY, Han HS, Kwon Y, Lee KS, Kim TH, et al. Breast cancer subtypes and survival in patients with brain metastases. Breast Cancer Res. 2008;10(1):R20.
84. Anders C, Deal AM, Abramson V, Liu MC, Storniolo AM, Carpenter JT, et al. TBCRC 018: phase II study of iniparib in combination with irinotecan to treat progressive triple negative breast cancer brain metastases. Breast Cancer Res Treat. 2014;146(3):557–66.
85. Karginova O, Siegel MB, Van Swearingen AE, Deal AM, Adamo B, Sambade MJ, et al. Efficacy of carboplatin alone and in combination with ABT888 in intracranial murine models of BRCA-mutated and BRCA-wild-type triple-negative breast cancer. Mol Cancer Ther. 2015;14(4):920–30.
86. Hoch U, Staschen CM, Johnson RK, Eldon MA. Nonclinical pharmacokinetics and activity of etirinotecan pegol (NKTR-102), a long-acting topoisomerase 1 inhibitor, in multiple cancer models. Cancer Chemother Pharmacol. 2014;74(6):1125–37.
87. Perez EA, Awada A, O'Shaughnessy J, Rugo HS, Twelves C, Im S-A, et al. Etirinotecan pegol (NKTR-102) versus treatment of physician's choice in women with advanced breast cancer previously treated with an anthracycline, a taxane, and capecitabine (BEACON): a randomised, open-label, multicentre, phase 3 trial. Lancet Oncol. 2015;16(15):1556–68.
88. Roodman GD. Mechanisms of bone metastasis. N Engl J Med. 2004;350(16):1655–64.
89. Van Poznak CH, Temin S, Yee GC, Janjan NA, Barlow WE, Biermann JS, et al. American Society of Clinical Oncology executive summary of the clinical practice guideline update on the role of bone-modifying agents in metastatic breast cancer. J Clin Oncol. 2011;29(9):1221–7.
90. Hortobagyi GN, Van Poznak C, Harker WG, Gradishar WJ, Chew H, Dakhil SR, et al. Continued treatment effect of zoledronic acid dosing every 12 vs 4 weeks in women with breast cancer metastatic to bone: the OPTIMIZE-2 randomized clinical trial. JAMA Oncol. 2017;3(7):906–12.

91. Perou CM, Sorlie T, Eisen MB, van de Rijn M, Jeffrey SS, Rees CA, et al. Molecular portraits of human breast tumours. Nature. 2000;406(6797):747–52.
92. Lehmann BD, Bauer JA, Chen X, Sanders ME, Chakravarthy AB, Shyr Y, et al. Identification of human triple-negative breast cancer subtypes and preclinical models for selection of targeted therapies. J Clin Invest. 2011;121(7):2750–67.
93. Prat A, Perou CM. Deconstructing the molecular portraits of breast cancer. Mol Oncol. 2011;5(1):5–23.
94. Shah SP, Roth A, Goya R, Oloumi A, Ha G, Zhao Y, et al. The clonal and mutational evolution spectrum of primary triple-negative breast cancers. Nature. 2012;486(7403):395–9.
95. Lehmann BD, Jovanovic B, Chen X, Estrada MV, Johnson KN, Shyr Y, et al. Refinement of triple-negative breast cancer molecular subtypes: implications for neoadjuvant chemotherapy selection. PLoS One. 2016;11(6):e0157368.
96. Ring BZ, Hout DR, Morris SW, Lawrence K, Schweitzer BL, Bailey DB, et al. Generation of an algorithm based on minimal gene sets to clinically subtype triple negative breast cancer patients. BMC Cancer. 2016;16(1):1–8.
97. The Cancer Genome Atlas Network. Comprehensive molecular portraits of human breast tumours. Nature. 2012;490(7418):61–70.

Molecular Profiling and Targeted Therapy for Triple-Negative Breast Cancer

9

April T. Swoboda and Rita Nanda

Clinical Pearls

- Triple-negative breast cancer is a heterogeneous disease with distinct molecular subtypes that correlate with response to therapy and clinical outcomes.
- Poly(ADP-ribose) polymerase inhibitors show efficacy as a single agent in *BRCA 1/2*-associated metastatic triple-negative breast cancer.
- Antiandrogen therapy shows clinical benefit in the androgen receptor subtype of triple-negative breast cancer.
- Checkpoint inhibitors, including anti-PD-1 and anti-PD-L1 antibodies, are demonstrating clinical activity in metastatic triple-negative breast cancer, and several studies are underway to further evaluate efficacy and understand biomarkers of response.

9.1 Molecular Profiling of Triple-Negative Breast Cancer

Triple-negative breast cancer (TNBC) is a heterogeneous disease with diverse histologic and molecular subtypes. Initial gene expression studies suggested that TNBC displayed primarily basal-like gene expression [1, 2]. When analyzed independently from hormone receptor-positive (HR+) and human epidermal growth factor receptor 2 (HER2)-positive breast cancers, triple-negative breast cancers exhibit distinct gene expression patterns that can be used to identify different TNBC subtypes [3].

A.T. Swoboda, MD • R. Nanda, MD (✉)
Section of Hematology/Oncology, The University of Chicago Medicine, Chicago, IL, USA
e-mail: april.swoboda@uchospitals.edu; rnanda@medicine.bsd.uchicago.edu

© Springer International Publishing AG 2018
A.R. Tan (ed.), *Triple-Negative Breast Cancer*,
https://doi.org/10.1007/978-3-319-69980-6_9

9.2   TNBCtype Classification

Several researchers have attempted to classify TNBC into molecular subtypes. Using gene expression analyses from 386 different tumors, Lehmann and colleagues initially identified six TNBC molecular subtypes (TNBCtype) with distinct biology and differential responses to chemotherapy [3]. These subtypes included basal-like 1 and basal-like 2 (BL1 and BL2), immunomodulatory (IM), mesenchymal (M), mesenchymal stem-like (MSL), and luminal androgen receptor (LAR). The BL1 subtype is characterized by elevated cell cycle and DNA damage response gene expression, while the BL2 subtype is characterized by increased growth factor signaling and myoepithelial markers. The IM subtype is enriched for genes involved in immune cell signaling, including immune antigens and cytokines, as well as core immune signal transduction pathways. The M and MSL subtypes share elevated expression of genes involved in epithelial-mesenchymal transition (EMT) and growth factor pathways. However, the MSL subtype has decreased expression of proliferation genes. The LAR subtype is characterized by an androgen receptor (AR) gene signature and high levels of luminal cytokeratin expression [3].

9.3   TNBCtype-4 Classification

The TNBCtype molecular subtypes were identified using surgical tumor specimens which contained significant amounts of normal tissue and stromal and immune components. To further examine the contribution of these non-tumor cells to the TNBC subtypes, Lehmann and colleagues used histopathological quantification, laser-capture microdissection, RNA isolation, and gene expression analysis on a panel of TNBC tumors and determined that transcripts in the previously described IM and MSL subtypes were contributed primarily from infiltrating lymphocytes and tumor-associated stromal cells, respectively. This led to a refinement of the original TNBCtype (BL1, BL2, IM, M, MSL, and LAR) to a TNBCtype-4 classification (BL1, BL2, M, and LAR) [4].

Lehmann and colleagues used the TNBCtype-4 classification to analyze 587 TNBC tumors with publicly available gene expression data [3] and 180 additional cases from The Cancer Genome Atlas (TCGA) [5]. When analyzed using the predictor analysis of microarray 50 (PAM50, by Prosigna), a 50-gene test that characterizes tumors by intrinsic subtype [6], the majority of BL1, BL2, and M tumors were basal-like, while the LAR subtype was enriched in the HER2 and luminal subtypes.

Histologically, BL1 tumors were primarily ductal carcinomas, while lobular carcinomas were almost exclusively of the LAR subtype, suggesting a role for AR signaling in lobular carcinoma. Medullary carcinomas, characterized by circumscribed pushing borders, dense peripheral lymphocytic infiltrate, and relatively favorable outcomes, were absent in the M subtype, consistent with its observed lack of tumor-infiltrating lymphocytes (TILs). Metaplastic breast cancers display striking diversity in morphology and were characterized by histological evidence of epithelial-mesenchymal transition (EMT) toward spindle, chondroid, osseous, and rhabdoid cell types. While PAM50 classified all the metaplastic tumors as basal-like, TNBCtype-4 subtyping could capture more subtle molecular differences and distinguish BL2 from M metaplastic tumors.

TNBCtype-4 molecular subtype correlated with a variety of clinicopathologic features. LAR tumors were associated with a lower grade than BL1 tumors ($P = 0.0003$). BL1 tumors were associated with a higher grade but a lower clinical stage at diagnosis compared to BL2 and LAR tumors (6%, 30%, 22% stage 3, respectively; $P = 0.0003$). Regional lymph node spread was more prevalent in the LAR subtype (47%) ($P = 0.0278$), compared to all other subtypes (34%) and the M subtype (21%), which had the lowest prevalence of regional nodal spread.

Metastatic patterns also varied by TNBCtype-4. The LAR subtype demonstrated a higher incidence of bone metastasis compared to all other subtypes (46% vs. 16%; $P = 0.0456$), while the M subtype displayed a higher frequency of lung metastasis compared to all others (46% vs. 25%; $P = 0.0388$). The predilection for the LAR subtype to metastasize to bone is consistent with the tissue tropism observed in other hormonally-regulated cancers and likely reflects unique tumor biology [7]. Overall survival (OS) and relapse-free survival (RFS) were significantly longer for BL1 patients, with near 60% RFS at 10 years.

9.4 Molecular Subtype and Response to Neoadjuvant Chemotherapy

Masuda et al. demonstrated a correlation between TNBCtype and response to anthracycline and taxane-based neoadjuvant chemotherapy (NACT) [8]. Pathologic complete response (pCR) was defined as the absence of residual invasive carcinoma in the breast and axillary lymph nodes upon histologic evaluation after receiving NACT (ypT0 or ypTis and ypN0). In their study, BL1 had the highest pCR rate (50%), while BL2 and LAR had the lowest (0% and 10%, respectively).

Lehmann and colleagues examined the same patient cohort using the refined TNBCtype-4 and found that subtyping did not result in significant differences ($P = 0.1074$) in pCR between the groups [4]. Compared to all other TNBC subtypes, however, the BL1 patients had a significantly higher rate of pCR (49% vs. 31%; $P = 0.0441$). The pCR incidence across the subtypes demonstrated similar trends as previous studies, with the BL1 subtype displaying the highest pCR rate and BL2 and LAR with the lowest rates.

Assessment of distant relapse-free survival (DRFS) by TNBCtype-4 stratification trended toward statistical significance ($P = 0.09$). The BL1 subtype, which had the highest incidence of pCR, had the longest DRFS interval with 72% of patient's relapse free at 7-year follow-up. In contrast, the BL2 subtype had the poorest outcome, with a median survival of 2.4 years compared to greater than 7 years for all TNBC patients.

To further study how TNBCtype-4 subtyping correlates with patient outcome, Lehmann and colleagues [4] combined multiple data sets with comparable classes of NACT. The combined cohort of 306 patients had an overall pCR rate of 21%. Patients with TNBC were significantly more likely to have a pCR than patients with non-TNBC (33% vs. 16%; $P = 0.0001$), and patients with PAM50 basal-like TNBC had a greater pCR rate than those with non-basal-like TNBC (36% vs. 20%; $P = 0.0175$). The rate of pCR for the BL2 subtype (18%) was far below the unselected TNBC population (33%) and slightly lower than the PAM50 non-basal-like TNBC subtype (20%). In contrast, the pCR rate for the BL1 subtype (41%) was higher than the rate for unselected TNBC (33%) and the PAM50 basal-like TNBC (36%).

While prospective studies are needed to validate these findings, these results suggest that molecular subtyping of patients with TNBC by TNBCtype-4 could identify patients who are less likely to respond to standard neoadjuvant chemotherapy and may therefore benefit from novel therapeutic approaches.

9.5   Other Molecular Classifications

Burstein and colleagues performed a similar gene expression analysis on a smaller cohort of 84 patients and identified four stable TNBC molecular phenotypes: luminal androgen receptor (AR; LAR), mesenchymal (MES), basal-like immunosuppressed (BLIS), and basal-like immune-activated (BLIA) [9]. These subtypes were characterized by distinct molecular profiles and clinical outcomes. As seen in the original TNBCtype classification [3], patients with TNBC enriched in immune-related genes had the best outcome [9]. There was overlap between the BL1 subtype with BLIA, the M subtype with BLIS, and the two LAR subtypes. While there are genomic alterations shared across all TNBC, individual molecular subtypes may be enriched in targetable somatic mutations, providing opportunities for preclinical and clinical investigation.

9.6   Targeted Therapy for Triple-Negative Breast Cancer

The standard of care treatment for TNBC in the neoadjuvant, adjuvant, and metastatic settings is chemotherapy. There are no targeted therapies currently approved by the US Food and Drug Administration (FDA) for the treatment of TNBC. Multiple novel targeted therapies and immunotherapies are currently under investigation.

9.6.1   Poly(ADP-ribose) Polymerase (PARP) Inhibitors

BRCA1 and *BRCA2* are tumor-suppressor genes that encode proteins involved in the repair of DNA double-strand breaks through the homologous recombination repair pathway [10, 11]. In contrast, members of the PARP family of enzymes, primarily PARP1 and PARP2, play a key role in the repair of DNA single-strand breaks through the base excision repair pathway [12, 13]. PARP inhibition in cells that lack functional *BRCA1* or *BRCA2* expression generates unrepaired DNA single-strand breaks, which accumulate and lead to obstruction and collapse of the replication fork, frequently resulting in DNA double-strand breaks and ultimately leading to cell death [14]. This exemplifies the concept of "synthetic lethality," which occurs when there is a lethal synergy between two otherwise nonlethal events [15].

9.6.1.1 BRCA-Associated Breast Cancer

Clinical trials conducted with PARP inhibitors have focused on patients with germline *BRCA 1/2* mutations, with promising results [16]. Olaparib is an oral PARP inhibitor approved by the FDA for treatment of patients with *BRCA1/2*-associated recurrent ovarian cancer. In a phase II trial of olaparib monotherapy in two sequential cohorts of *BRCA*-mutated advanced TNBC, an overall response rate (ORR) of 54% (7 of 13 patients) was seen in the cohort treated at 400 mg po twice daily, compared to an ORR of 25% (4 of 16 patients) in the cohort treated at 100 mg po twice daily [17]. Another phase II trial of olaparib monotherapy in *BRCA*-mutated advanced breast cancer had an ORR of 13.3% (95% CI, 3.8–30.7) for patients with ER-negative disease (4 of 30), which might be attributed to the inclusion of a more heavily pretreated population as these patients were required to have received at least three prior lines of chemotherapy [18]. The OlympiAD trial was a randomized, open-label phase III trial designed to compare olaparib monotherapy at 300 mg po twice daily with standard single-agent chemotherapy of physician's choice (capecitabine, eribulin, or vinorelbine in 21-day cycles) among 302 patients with HER2-negative metastatic breast cancer and a germline *BRCA* mutation [19]. The ORR in the olaparib group was approximately double that of the standard therapy group (59.9% vs. 28.8%), and the median progression-free survival (PFS) was significantly longer in the olaparib group than in the standard therapy group (7.0 vs. 4.2 months; hazard ratio 0.58; 95% CI, 0.43–0.80; $P < 0.001$). Time to onset of response, an important consideration for symptomatic patients or those with rapidly progressing disease, was similar in the two groups. Olaparib was well tolerated, with fewer grade 3 and greater adverse events (AEs) and AEs leading to discontinuation than occurred with standard therapy. The most common treatment-related AE in the olaparib group was grade 1 or 2 nausea, and the most common ≥ grade 3 AE was anemia. A randomized, double-blind, placebo-controlled phase III trial called OlympiA is currently investigating the use of olaparib as adjuvant monotherapy for up to 12 months in high-risk TNBC patients with germline *BRCA1/2* mutations who have completed definitive local treatment and at least six cycles of neoadjuvant or adjuvant chemotherapy [20].

Veliparib, another oral PARP inhibitor under investigation for the treatment of *BRCA*-mutated breast cancer, has shown single-agent activity, as well as activity in combination with carboplatin or temozolomide (TMZ) [21, 22]. In a phase II study of TMZ and veliparib in 41 patients with metastatic breast cancer, patients received veliparib 40 mg po twice a day on days 1–7 and TMZ 150 mg/m² po daily on days 1–5, on a 28-day cycle. After a higher than expected grade 4 thrombocytopenia was observed, the dose of veliparib was reduced to 30 mg twice a day. Activity was observed only in patients with known *BRCA1/2* mutations, with a response rate of 50% (4/8). Based on this observation, the investigators enrolled an expansion cohort of 20 additional patients with *BRCA1/2* mutations. Combined with the initial cohort of 8 known mutation carriers from the original 41 patients, the total response rate was 25% (7/28) with a clinical benefit rate of 50% (7 PR, 7 SD) [23]. Results from both arms of a larger randomized phase II trial of veliparib with temozolomide or carboplatin/paclitaxel vs. placebo with carboplatin/paclitaxel in *BRCA1/2*-mutated metastatic breast cancer were reported at the 2016 San Antonio Breast Cancer Symposium (SABCS) [24–26]. Veliparib and carboplatin/paclitaxel (V+C/P) demonstrated a statistically significant improvement in ORR compared to the placebo and carboplatin/paclitaxel (Plc+C/P) arm (77.8% vs. 61.3%; $P = 0.027$). There were trends toward improved PFS (14.1 vs. 12.3 months) and OS (28.5 vs. 25.0 months) in the V+C/P vs. Plc+C/P arms, respectively; however, these were not statistically significant. The most common treatment-related adverse events (TRAEs) across both treatment arms were neutropenia, thrombocytopenia, and nausea, but patients reported significant improvements in fatigue, pain, and insomnia (all $P < 0.05$) with V+C/P compared to Plc+C/P [26]. In the analysis of veliparib and TMZ (V+TMZ) vs. Plc+C/P, median PFS, median OS (interim), and ORR were inferior in the V+TMZ arm (PFS 7.4 vs. 12.3 months, OS 19.1 vs. 25.0 months, and ORR 28.6% vs. 61.3%) [25]. V+TMZ was well tolerated, with less neutropenia, alopecia, and peripheral neuropathy observed compared to the Plc+C/P arm. The most common grade ≥ 3 AEs were thrombocytopenia and neutropenia. Phase III trials evaluating other PARP inhibitors in *BRCA*-mutated metastatic breast cancer are ongoing, including niraparib in BRAVO [27] and talazoparib in EMBRACA [28].

9.6.1.2 Sporadic Triple-Negative Breast Cancer and BRCAness

The most robust evidence for the benefit of PARP inhibitors in breast cancer has been demonstrated in patients harboring germline *BRCA1* and *BRCA2* mutations. While the prevalence of *BRCA1/2* mutations in TNBC is approximately 10%, some sporadic TNBCs share molecular features of *BRCA*-mutant tumors, a concept known as "BRCAness" [29, 30]. As described by Lord and Ashworth, based on our current understanding of cancer genetics, genomics, and mechanisms of DNA repair, BRCAness represents a phenocopy of *BRCA1* or *BRCA2* mutations. It describes a phenotype in which a homologous recombination repair defect exists in a tumor in the absence of a germline *BRCA1/2* mutation [31]. As such, these sporadic TNBCs may respond to similar therapeutic approaches, including PARP inhibition.

The neoadjuvant, phase II, multicenter I-SPY2 trial (Investigation of Serial Studies to Predict Your Therapeutic Response through Imaging and Molecular Analysis 2) is an ongoing study evaluating multiple experimental arms, including the addition of veliparib and carboplatin to standard weekly paclitaxel followed by doxorubicin and cyclophosphamide, in stage II–III breast cancer patients regardless of *BRCA*-mutation status [32]. The trial utilizes an adaptive randomization algorithm based on biomarker "signatures" to assign patients to treatment arms that are performing well for patients who share their biomarker signature; the primary endpoint is pCR (ypT0/N0 or ypTis/N0). The estimated pCR rates in the TNBC population were 51% (95% Bayesian probability interval [PI], 36–66) vs. 26% (95% PI, 9–43) in the veliparib/carboplatin and control groups, respectively. Based on these results, the veliparib/carboplatin arm "graduated" to a randomized phase III trial. The I-SPY2 trial was not designed to evaluate the individual contributions of veliparib and carboplatin, but this was subsequently investigated in the phase III Brightness trial comparing the efficacy of carboplatin or veliparib plus carboplatin in combination with standard neoadjuvant chemotherapy in patients with early-stage TNBC [33]. The result of this trial was presented at the 2017 American Society of Clinical Oncology Annual Meeting, and Geyer and colleagues found that while the addition of veliparib and carboplatin did increase the pCR rate as compared to control (53.2% vs. 31.0%, $P < 0.001$), the combination did not increase pCR rates as compared to the addition of carboplatin alone (53.2% vs. 57.5%, $P = 0.36$), demonstrating that the improvement in pCR was due to carboplatin, without any contribution from the veliparib.

9.7   Androgen Receptor Antagonists

Interest in targeting the androgen receptor (AR) in TNBC began with the observation that a group of TNBCs, referred to as the luminal androgen receptor (LAR) subtype, was characterized by high AR expression, luminal gene expression pattern, and dependence on hormone signaling [3]. While AR can be expressed in other molecular subtypes of TNBC, the LAR subtype has the highest levels of AR expression [34], with distinct clinical features and outcome. Loibl and colleagues reported that AR-negative tumors were more likely to achieve a pCR with neoadjuvant docetaxel/doxorubicin/cyclophosphamide (TAC) chemotherapy than AR-positive (AR+) tumors (25.4% vs. 12.8%, $P = <0.0001$) [35]. However, despite their decreased responsiveness to neoadjuvant chemotherapy, TNBC patients with AR+ tumors had significantly better DFS and OS than TNBC patients with AR-negative tumors. Masuda and colleagues reported similar findings, with a decreased pCR rate among the LAR subtype (10%) of TNBC compared to all TNBC (28%) [8]. These findings suggested that AR+ TNBC does not receive the same benefit from standard chemotherapy as AR-negative TNBC.

9.7.1   Bicalutamide

Bicalutamide is an oral, nonsteroidal, AR antagonist approved by the US FDA for use in combination with luteinizing hormone-releasing hormone (LHRH) analogs for the treatment of metastatic prostate cancer. Translational Breast Cancer Research Consortium (TBCRC) 011, an open-label, single-arm, phase II study of bicalutamide, was the first clinical trial to report activity of targeting AR in advanced AR+

TNBC [36]. Of note, at the time of study accrual, ASCO/CAP guidelines had not yet decreased the threshold for defining ER and PR positivity to its current level of ≥1% [37]. Of the 424 patients screened, 51 (12%) were AR+, defined as immunohistochemistry (IHC) >10% nuclear staining, and the final study population included 26 patients. Treatment with bicalutamide 150 mg po once daily led to a clinical benefit rate (CBR) of 19% (95% CI, 7–39%), defined as the total number of patients with a complete response (CR), partial response (PR), or stable disease (SD) for >6 months. Median PFS was 12 weeks (95% CI, 11–22 weeks), and the number of cycles received ranged from 2 to 84. Bicalutamide was well tolerated. The most common TRAEs were fatigue, hot flashes, limb edema, aspartate aminotransferase (AST) elevation, and alkaline aminotransferase (ALT) elevation. The study met its primary endpoints for efficacy and established the androgen receptor as a relevant target in AR+ TNBC.

9.7.2   Abiraterone Acetate

Abiraterone acetate (AA) is a selective, irreversible, and potent inhibitor of 17-[α]-hydroxylase/17,20-lyase (CYP17) enzymatic activity and is commonly used in castration-resistant prostate cancer (CRPC). The open-label, single-arm phase II UCBG 12-1 trial of abiraterone acetate had results similar to TBCRC 011, with 37.6% of TNBC patients demonstrating AR positivity (IHC ≥10%) and a 6-month CBR of 20% (95% CI, 7.7–38.6%) [38]. Patients received 1000 mg of AA at four 250 mg tablets po once a day. For the 30 evaluable patients, ORR was 6.7% (95% CI, 0.8–22.1%), and median PFS was 2.8 months (95% CI, 1.7–5.4%). The most common TRAEs were fatigue, hypertension, hypokalemia, and nausea and were mostly grade 1 or 2.

9.7.3   Enzalutamide

In the largest study of an AR inhibitor in TNBC, enzalutamide, a potent oral inhibitor approved for use in men with metastatic CRPC, has been evaluated in an open-label phase II trial by Traina and colleagues [39]. Enzalutamide at 160 mg po daily was tested in the 118 patient intent-to-treat (ITT) population with advanced AR+ TNBC, defined in this study as any AR expression by IHC (> 0%). The evaluable population (n = 75) consisted of a subset of patients with AR IHC expression ≥10% and at least one post-baseline tumor assessment. The primary endpoint was clinical benefit (CR, PR, or SD) at 16 weeks (CBR16) in evaluable patients. In the evaluable population, the CBR16 was 35% and median PFS was 14.7 weeks. This trial reported the first ever objective responses with androgen-directed therapy in TNBC, with a confirmed complete or partial response rate of 8%. The most common TRAEs were fatigue, nausea, decreased appetite, diarrhea, and hot flush. Fatigue was the only AE grade ≥ 3 in ≥5% of patients.

Traina and colleagues developed an androgen-driven genomic signature (PREDICT AR, now known as Dx), classifying patients as Dx-positive (Dx+) or Dx-negative (Dx−) [40]. The 47% of patients that were Dx+ had a doubling in PFS (16 weeks vs. 8 weeks) compared to Dx− patients. At median follow-up of 28 months for all patients, median OS in the unselected population was 13 months (95% CI, 8–18) [41]. In the Dx+ subgroup, median OS was 20 months (95% CI, 13–29) vs. 8 months (95% CI, 5–11) in the Dx− subgroup. In patients with no more than one prior line of therapy, median OS in the Dx+ subgroup was 29 months, longer than that of unselected historic controls, compared to 10 months in the Dx− subgroup.

9.8 Glucocorticoid Receptor Antagonists

The glucocorticoid receptor (GR) is overexpressed in up to 50% of invasive breast cancers [42]. By regulating the transcription of genes encoding antiapoptotic pathways, GR activation plays a critical role in promoting cell survival under otherwise apoptosis-inducing conditions, such as chemotherapy [43, 44]. In contrast to ER+ breast cancers, in which GR expression is correlated with improved outcome, high tumor GR mRNA expression in early-stage ER-negative cancers is associated with shorter RFS, regardless of whether patients receive chemotherapy, suggesting a role in resistance to chemotherapy [45].

Based on preclinical data demonstrating that pretreatment with a GR antagonist, mifepristone, increases the cytotoxicity of chemotherapy in GR-positive (GR+) TNBC [44], a randomized phase I trial evaluated nab-paclitaxel with or without mifepristone in advanced breast cancer patients [46]. Patients were treated with intravenous (IV) weekly nab-paclitaxel on days 1, 8, and 15 of each 28 day cycle at a starting dose of 100 mg/m^2. Mifepristone was administered orally for two consecutive days, starting 1 day prior to each nab-paclitaxel infusion at a starting dose of 300 mg po per day. Of the nine patients enrolled, six patients were found to be GR+ by IHC (>10% nuclear GR staining), all of whom were also triple-negative. Of note, two of these patients initially presented with ER+ disease, but tumors had converted to TNBC at the time of disease recurrence. Among the six patients in the GR+ subgroup, there were two CRs, two PRs, one SD, and one PD. The GR-negative subgroup had one PR and two PDs. Neutropenia occurred at both of the studied nab-paclitaxel doses but was easily managed with dose reduction and/or growth factor administration. Based on these promising results, a randomized phase II trial of nab-paclitaxel with or without mifepristone in GR+ TNBC patients is underway.

The safety and tolerability of mifepristone in combination with carboplatin and gemcitabine for advanced breast and ovarian cancer were established in another phase I clinical trial [47]. Eighteen of the thirty-one patients enrolled had breast cancer. Of the 13 TNBC patients that were evaluable for a response, two had a CR, one had a PR, six had SD, and four had PD. Again, the most common dose-limiting toxicity (DLT) was neutropenia that was easily managed with the institution of pro-phylactic granulocyte-colony stimulating factor (G-CSF). Correlative studies are ongoing to identify predictive biomarkers of response to this combination.

9.9   Immunotherapy

Programmed death receptor-1 (PD-1) is an inhibitory transmembrane protein expressed on T cells, B cells, and NK cells; its ligands are programmed death-ligand 1 (PD-L1), also known as B7-H1, and programmed death-ligand 2 (PD-L2), also known as B7-H2 [48]. While PD-L1 is expressed on the surface of multiple types of cells, including many tumor and hematopoietic cells, PD-L2 is primarily expressed on hematopoietic cells [49]. The PD-1/PD-L1/2 interaction directly inhibits apopto-sis of the tumor cell, promotes peripheral T effector cell exhaustion, and promotes conversion of T effector cells to T regulatory (Treg) cells [50, 51]. PD-1 and PD-L1/L2 are generally upregulated in the context of pro-effector cytokines (such as IFN-γ) secreted by CD8+ tumor-infiltrating lymphocytes (TIL), highlighting their role as "immune checkpoints" functioning as a physiologic brake on unrestrained cytotoxic T effector function [52, 53]. Targeting the PD-1/PD-L1 axis with immune check-point blockade should, therefore, enhance anticancer immunity.

9.9.1   Pembrolizumab

Pembrolizumab (MK-3475) is a highly selective, humanized immunoglobulin (Ig) G4-κ monoclonal antibody specific for PD-1, currently FDA-approved for use in metastatic melanoma, non-small cell lung cancer, squamous cell carcinoma of the head and neck (SCCHN), urothelial carcinoma, and classical Hodgkin lymphoma. It received accelerated approval for adult and pediatric patients with unresectable or metastatic microsatellite instability-high (MSI-H) or mismatch repair-deficient (dMMR) solid tumors that have progressed following prior treatment and who have no satisfactory alternative treatment options. This landmark approval marks the first tumor tissue/site-agnostic indication granted by the FDA, with approval based on a common biomarker rather than the location of the body where the tumor originated.

KEYNOTE-012 was a phase Ib multicohort study of single-agent pembroli-zumab 10 mg/kg intravenously every 2 weeks in patients with advanced PD-L1-positive (PD-L1+) solid tumors, including TNBC, gastric cancer, urothelial cancer, and head and neck cancer [54]. PD-L1 positivity was defined as PD-L1 expression in stroma or ≥1% of tumor cells by IHC using the Merck 22C3 antibody. The TNBC cohort enrolled 32 women with recurrent or metastatic PD-L1+ TNBC. Of the 111 patients screened for PD-L1 expression, 58.6% had PD-L1+ tumors. Median age was 50.5 years in this heavily pretreated population. Patients had received a median of two prior lines of systemic therapy for metastatic disease, with 46.9% of patients having received at least three lines of therapy. Among the 27 patients who were evaluable for antitumor activity, the primary endpoint of ORR was 18.5% (1 CR, 4 PRs), with a median time to response of 17.9 weeks (range, 7.3–32.4 weeks). Durable responses were observed, with the median duration of response not yet reached (range, 15.0 to ≥47.3 weeks), including three responders remaining on treatment for ≥12 months. The most common TRAEs were arthralgias, fatigue, myalgias, and nausea, which were mild and similar to those observed in other tumor cohorts. Five patients (15.6%) had grade ≥ 3 AEs, and there was one treatment-related death due to disseminated intravascular coagulation.

The phase II KEYNOTE-086 study evaluated pembrolizumab monotherapy in two cohorts: previously treated metastatic TNBC regardless of PD-L1 expression (Cohort A) and first-line PD-L1+ metastatic TNBC (Cohort B) [55, 56]. Of the 170 patients enrolled in cohort A, (median age 53.5 years; range, 28–85 years), 43.5% had ≥3 prior lines of therapy, and 61.8% had PD-L1+ tumors [55]. Patients received pembrolizumab 200 mg intravenously every 3 weeks. After a median follow-up of 10.9 months, nine patients (5.3%) remained on pembrolizumab. Primary endpoint of overall ORR was 4.7% (95% CI, 2.3–9.2%). ORR was the same regardless of PD-L1 expression (4.8% in PD-L1+ patients vs. 4.7% in PD-L1-negative patients). Median duration of response (DOR) was 6.3 months (range, 1.2+ to 10.3+ months). Median PFS and OS were 2.0 months (95% CI, 1.9–2.0) and 8.9 months (95% CI, 7.2–11.2 months), with 6-month rates of 12.3% and 69%, respectively. TRAEs of any grade and grade ≥ 3 occurred in 60% and 12.4% of patients, respectively. There were no deaths due to AEs and 4% of patients discontinued pembrolizumab due to TRAEs.

Of the first 52 patients enrolled in cohort B of KEYNOTE-086 for first-line treatment of metastatic TNBC, median age was 53 years (range, 26–80 years), and 87% had received prior (neo)adjuvant therapy [56]. After a median follow-up of 7.0 months (range, 4.4–12.5 months), 15 (29%) patients remained on pembrolizumab. The primary endpoint was safety. TRAEs occurred in 37 (71%) patients. The most common were fatigue (31%), nausea (15%), and diarrhea (13%). Four (8%) patients experienced grade ≥ 3 TRAEs: back pain, fatigue, hyponatremia, hypotension, and migraine ($n = 1$ each). No patients died or discontinued pembrolizumab due to an AE. ORR was 23.1% (95% CI, 14–36%). The best overall response was CR in 4%, PR in 19%, SD in 17%, PD in 58%, and not assessed in 2%. Median time to response was 8.7 weeks (range, 8.1–17.7 weeks), and median DOR was 8.4 months (range, 2.1+ to 8.4 months), with 8 (67%) responses ongoing at data cutoff. Median PFS was 2.1 months (95% CI, 2.0–3.9 months), with estimated 6-month PFS rate 28%. A randomized phase III trial of pembrolizumab monotherapy compared to physician's choice of single-agent chemotherapy (capecitabine, eribulin, gemcitabine, or vinorelbine) in metastatic TNBC is ongoing (KEYNOTE-119; NCT02555657) [57].

A phase Ib/II study evaluated pembrolizumab in combination with eribulin in patients with metastatic TNBC unselected for PD-L1 expression [58]. A phase Ib included a safety run-in cohort in which ≥6 patients received intravenous eribulin mesylate 1.4 mg/m^2 on days 1 and 8 and IV pembrolizumab 200 mg on day 1 of a 21-day cycle, which was used as the recommended phase II dose (RP2D). An interim analysis of the first 39 enrolled patients ($n = 7$, phase Ib; $n = 32$, phase II) was presented at the 2016 SABCS. The median age was 53 years (range, 32–80 years), and the study included patients previously treated with 0–2 lines of chemotherapy in the metastatic setting. Primary endpoints were determination of safety and tolerability (phase Ib) and evaluation of ORR (phase II). Secondary endpoints included evaluation of PFS, OS, and DOR. No DLTs were observed in phase Ib. The most common TRAEs were fatigue, nausea, peripheral neuropathy, neutropenia, and alopecia, with the most frequent grade ≥ 3 AEs being neutropenia and fatigue. Median duration of treatment was 3.9 months for eribulin (range, 1.0–8.3 months) and 3.7 months for pembrolizumab (range, 0.8–9.0 months). ORR was 33.3% (1 CR, 12 PRs). In stratum 1, which consisted of patients with no prior lines of treatment in the metastatic setting, ORR was 41.2% (95% CI, 19.3–62.8%) vs. 27.3% (95% CI, 11.3–46.4%) in stratum 2 (1–2 prior lines of treatment). PD-L1 status did not predict response to treatment. ORR was 29.4% (95% CI, 11.1–51.1%) in the PD-L1+ patients vs. 33.3% (95% CI, 14.1–54.6%) in PD-L1-negative patients. Overall, the combination of pembrolizumab and eribulin demonstrated activity in metastatic TNBC, and AEs observed with the combination were comparable to those observed historically with either treatment as monotherapy. A phase III clinical trial to evaluate the safety and efficacy of pembrolizumab in combination with chemotherapy (either paclitaxel, nab-paclitaxel, or carboplatin/gemcitabine) in the first-line treatment of metastatic TNBC is currently underway (KEYNOTE-355; NCT02819518).

Pembrolizumab has also been investigated in the neoadjuvant setting in the I-SPY2 trial, in which 69 patients were adaptively randomized to the pembrolizumab arm (pembrolizumab in combination with paclitaxel, followed by doxorubicin plus cyclophosphamide) and 180 patients were randomized to the control arm [59]. The addition of pembrolizumab to chemotherapy significantly increased the estimated pCR rates in all biomarker signatures studied (HR+/HER2-negative, TNBC, and all HER2-negative). The estimated pCR rates in the TNBC population were 60% in the pembrolizumab group (95% Bayesian probability interval [PI], 43–78%) vs. 20.0% (95% PI, 6–33%) in the control group. In the HR+ group, the estimated pCR rate was 34% (95% PI, 19–48%) in the pembrolizumab group vs. 13% (95% PI, 3–24%) in the control group. Six patients who received pembrolizumab experienced grade 3 primary or secondary adrenal insufficiency. Five of these patients presented after completion of AC (10–12 weeks after completion), and one presented 37 days after starting pembrolizumab. Nine patients had grade 1–2 thyroid abnormalities; one had grade 3 hypothyroidism. The most common grade ≥ 3 AEs in the pembrolizumab arm were diarrhea, febrile neutropenia, fatigue, anemia, and nausea. Based on Bayesian predictive probability of success in a confirmatory phase III trial, pembrolizumab "graduated" from the I-SPY2 trial for all signatures in which it was tested (TNBC, all HER2-negative, and HR+/HER2-negative). A randomized phase III neoadjuvant trial is accruing clinical stage IIA to IIIB TNBC patients who are candidates for potentially curative surgery. Randomization is to pembrolizumab or placebo with weekly paclitaxel and carboplatin (weekly or every

3 weeks) for four cycles followed by pembrolizumab or placebo plus doxorubicin (epirubicin can be substituted) and cyclophosphamide for four cycles as neoadjuvant therapy prior to surgery, which is then followed by nine cycles of pembrolizumab or placebo every 3 weeks as adjuvant therapy postsurgery (KEYNOTE-522; NCT03036488). The primary endpoint is pCR.

9.9.2 Atezolizumab

Atezolizumab (MPDL3280A) is a high-affinity, engineered, fully human IgG_1 monoclonal antibody that inhibits the interaction of PD-L1 with PD-1 and B7.1 (CD80), both of which are negative regulators of T lymphocyte activation [60]. Because PD-L1 is expressed on activated T cells, atezolizumab was engineered with a modification in the Fc domain that eliminates antibody-dependent cellular cytotoxicity (ADCC) at clinically relevant doses, thus preventing the depletion of T cells expressing PD-L1 [61]. It is FDA-approved for use in metastatic urothelial carcinoma and non-small cell lung cancer.

A phase Ia study evaluated the safety and efficacy of atezolizumab monotherapy in multiple disease-specific cohorts, including a cohort of 115 metastatic TNBC patients [62]. The TNBC cohort initially enrolled patients with PD-L1+ disease but was later amended to include patients with PD-L1-negative disease. Among prescreened patients, 63% had PD-L1+ tumors, defined as those containing ≥5% PD-L1+ tumor-infiltrating lymphocytes (TILs) using the SP142 antibody. Median age was 53 years (range, 29–82 years), and the population was heavily pretreated, with 58% of patients having received ≥3 systemic therapies in the metastatic setting. Patients received atezolizumab intravenously at 15 mg/kg, 20 mg/kg, or 1200 mg flat dose every 3 weeks. ORR in the 112 evaluable patients was 10% (95% CI, 5–17%), with median DOR 21.1 months (range, 2.8–26.5+ months) and median PFS 1.4 months (95% CI, 1.3–1.6 months). Three patients initially classified as having PD appeared to have had pseudoprogression, with evidence of ongoing clinical benefit and durable regression of target lesions despite the appearance of new lesions [63]. There was a marked difference in ORR depending on the line of treatment. ORR in patients previously untreated for metastatic disease was 26% (95% CI, 9–51%), compared to 4% in the second-line setting (95% CI, 0–18%) and 8% in patients who had received three or more lines of therapy (95% CI, 3–17%). Median OS at median follow-up of 15.2 months in all patients was 9.3 months (95% CI, 7.0–12.6 months). OS rates were 41% at 1 year (95% CI, 31–51%) and 22% at both 2 and 3 years (95% CI, 12–32%). Remarkably, OS for the 11 patients with an objective response (CR or PR) was 100% at 2 years. TRAEs were frequent (observed in 63% of patients). The most common were pyrexia, fatigue, and nausea, which were typically grade 1–2 and easily managed. About 11% of patients experienced grade ≥ 3 TRAEs, and there were two treatment-related deaths as assessed by the investigators (pulmonary hypertension and death not otherwise specified in a hospitalized patient).

The combination of atezolizumab 800 mg IV on days 1 and 15 and nab-paclitaxel 125 mg/m^2 on days 1, 8, and 15 of a 28-day cycle was evaluated for safety and clinical activity in a phase Ib study of patients with metastatic TNBC unselected for PD-L1 expression [64]. There were 32 patients enrolled. Median age was 55.5 years (range, 32–84 years), and patients could have received zero to three prior lines of therapy. At time of data cutoff, confirmed ORR was 38% (95% CI, 21–56%) in the 32 patients evaluable for efficacy. Two additional patients had pseudoprogression; they developed new lesions and were scored as PD based on RECIST (Response Evaluation Criteria in Solid Tumors), but had partial responses in target lesions and remained on treatment with prolonged biologic response. In the PD-L1+ cohort, ORR was 36% (95% CI, 11–69%) compared to 30% (95% CI, 7–65%) in the PD-L1-negative cohort. Grade 3 or 4 hematologic AEs was observed in 56% of patients; however, these were manageable and did not require treatment discontinuation. No DLT or treatment-related deaths occurred. Based on these results, the combination of atezolizumab and nab-paclitaxel is currently being investigated in the IMpassion130 trial (NCT02425891), a phase III randomized, double-blind, placebo-controlled study for the first-line treatment of patients with metastatic TNBC [65].

9.9.3 Avelumab

Avelumab (MSB0010718C) is a fully human anti-PD-L1 IgG$_1$-κ monoclonal antibody given intravenously that is currently FDA-approved for use in advanced urothelial carcinoma and Merkel cell carcinoma. In the phase Ib JAVELIN solid tumor trial, avelumab 10 mg/kg IV given every 2 weeks was investigated in locally advanced or metastatic breast cancer refractory to standard of care therapy [66]. Patients were unselected for PD-L1 expression or breast cancer subtype. A total of 168 patients were enrolled, with median age 55 years (range, 31–81 years). The population was heavily pretreated, with 52.4% of patients having had ≥3 prior lines of therapy, and 58 of 168 patients (34.5%) had TNBC. The ORR for the entire cohort was 4.8% (95% CI, 2.1–9.2%), with 1 CR and 7 PRs; 5 of the 8 responses were ongoing at the time of data cutoff. Stable disease was observed in 39 patients (23.2%) for an overall DCR of 28%. In the TNBC subgroup ($n = 58$), there were five PRs for an ORR of 8.6% (95% CI, 2.9–19.0%). Among TNBC patients with ≥10% PD-L1+ immune cells within the tumor, the so-called immune cell "hotspots," 44.4% (4 of 9) had response to therapy (PR). TRAEs were observed in 71.4% of patients, and the most common were fatigue, nausea, and infusion-related reactions. Grade ≥ 3 TRAEs occurred in 14.3% of patients and included fatigue, anemia, increased gamma-glutamyl transferase (GGT), autoimmune hepatitis, and arthralgias. There were two treatment-related deaths, from acute liver failure and respiratory distress.

Numerous additional studies of PD-1/PD-L1 inhibitors in combination with chemotherapy, targeted therapies, radiotherapy, and other immune checkpoint inhibitors are undergoing evaluation in metastatic TNBC patients.

9.10   PI3K-AKT-mTOR Inhibitors

The phosphatidylinositol-4,5-bisphosphate 3-kinase (PI3K)-AKT-mechanistic target of rapamycin (mTOR) pathway is an important intracellular signaling pathway that plays a critical role in carcinogenesis by promoting cell survival and growth [67, 68]. PI3K activation phosphorylates and activates AKT, the central node of the pathway, which then translocates to the cell membrane and can have downstream effects, such as the phosphorylation and regulation of various cellular proteins, including mTOR complex 1 (mTORC1) [68, 69]. Genomic analysis of TNBC has identified a subgroup with genetic activation of the PI3K/AKT pathway through multiple mechanisms, including alterations in *PTEN* and activating mutations in *PIK3CA* or *AKT1* [5]. As such, the three major nodes of this pathway represent promising therapeutic targets.

As part of the neoadjuvant I-SPY2 clinical trial, MK-2206, an allosteric AKT inhibitor, was evaluated in combination with weekly paclitaxel 80 mg/m^2 weekly for 12 weeks followed by doxorubicin 60 mg/m^2 and cyclophosphamide 600 mg/m^2 given every 2–3 weeks for four cycles versus chemotherapy alone [70]. The I-SPY2 trial involves a novel adaptive trial design based on Bayesian predictive probability that a biological regimen will be shown to be statistically superior to standard therapy in an equally randomized 300 patient confirmatory trial. Regimens that have a high Bayesian-predictive probability of showing superiority in at least 1 of 10 predefined signatures graduate from the trial. Regimens are dropped for futility if they show a low predictive probability of showing superiority over standard therapy in all ten signatures. MK-2206 graduated in the TNBC signature with an estimated pathologic complete response rate of 46.7% in the combination arm compared to 26.1% in the concurrent control arm. MK-2206 plus standard neoadjuvant chemotherapy was found to have a 98.6% chance of being superior to the control and an 82.7% likelihood of success in a phase III trial, and therefore met criteria for graduation in the TNBC signature.

The phase II randomized, double-blind, placebo-controlled LOTUS trial evaluated first-line treatment of metastatic TNBC with paclitaxel alone or in combination with ipatasertib [71]. Patients received intravenous paclitaxel 80 mg/m^2 on days 1, 8, and 15 with either oral ipatasertib 400 mg or placebo once a day on days 1–21 of a 28-day cycle. The ipatasertib and placebo arms each had 62 patients, and patients were classified into prespecified groups based on tumors with PTEN-low expression (IHC 0 in >50% of tumor cells using the Ventana IHC assay, clone SP218) or *PIK3CA/AKT1/PTEN* alteration assessed by Foundation One next-generation sequencing (NGS). Of the 101 assessable IHC samples, 48 (48%) were classified as PTEN-low, while 42 of the 103 (41%) samples assessed by NGS had *PIK3CA/AKT1/PTEN* alterations. Median follow-up was 10.4 months (interquartile range [IQR], 6.5–14.1 months) in the ipatasertib group and 10.2 months (IQR 6.0–13.6 months) in the placebo group. Median PFS in the ITT population was 6.2 months (95% CI, 3.8–9.0 months) in the ipatasertib group vs. 4.9 months (95% CI, 3.6–5.4 months) in the placebo group (stratified HR 0.60, 95% CI, 0.37–0.98; $P = 0.037$). In the 48 patients with PTEN-low tumors, median PFS was 6.2 months

(95% CI, 3.6–9.1 months) with ipatasertib vs. 3.7 months (95% CI, 1.9–7.3 months) with placebo (stratified HR 0.59, 95% CI, 0.26–1.32; $P = 0.18$). Prespecified subgroup analysis of the *PIK3CA/AKT1/PTEN*-altered tumors showed median PFS of 9.0 months (95% CI, 4.6-not assessable) with ipatasertib vs. 4.9 months (95% CI, 3.6–6.3 months) with placebo (non-stratified HR 0.44, 95% CI, 0.20–0.99; log-rank $P = 0.041$). The most common ≥ grade 3 TRAEs in the ipatasertib and placebo arms, respectively, were diarrhea (23% vs. 0%), neutrophil count decreased (8% vs. 6%), and neutropenia (10% vs. 2%). Overall, AEs were manageable and reversible. No treatment-related deaths occurred in the ipatasertib arm, while one occurred in the placebo arm. Serious AEs were reported in 28% of patients in the ipatasertib group vs. 15% in the placebo group. While the increase in median PFS was modest in the ITT and PTEN-low populations, improvement in median PFS was more pronounced in the predefined subgroup of patients with *PIK3CA/AKT1/PTEN*-altered tumors. A phase II randomized, placebo-controlled study (FAIRLANE trial; NCT02301988) is assessing the addition of ipatasertib to paclitaxel in the neoadjuvant triple-negative setting.

9.11 Antibody-Drug Conjugates

9.11.1 IMMU-132

Trop-2, a glycoprotein overexpressed in many carcinomas, including TNBC, is associated with a poor prognosis [72]. It plays a multifunctional cellular role, including acting as a calcium signal transducer that drives tumor growth. Sacituzumab govitecan (IMMU-132) is an anti-Trop-2/SN-38 antibody-drug conjugate (ADC) made from a humanized anti-Trop-2 monoclonal antibody (hRS7) conjugated with SN-38, the potent active metabolite of irinotecan [73–76], a topoisomerase I inhibitor that causes DNA double-strand breaks leading to apoptosis [77].

Bardia and colleagues evaluated IMMU-132 in a single-arm, multicenter phase II trial in patients with previously treated metastatic TNBC [78]. Trop-2 expression was not required for enrollment, but 88% of tumor specimens stained for Trop-2 by IHC assay were found to be moderately to strongly positive. Patients received 10 mg/kg intravenously on days 1 and 8 of a 21-day cycle; the primary endpoints were safety and ORR. In 69 patients who had received a median of five prior therapies (range, 1–12) since their metastatic diagnosis, the confirmed ORR was 30% (PR, $n = 19$; CR, $n = 2$) and the CBR (CR + PR + SD ≥6 months) was 46%. Median PFS was 6.0 months (95% CI, 5.0–7.3 months), and median OS was 16.6 months (95% CI, 11.1–20.6 months). Grade ≥ 3 AEs occurred in 41% of patients, the most common being neutropenia (39%), leukopenia (16%), anemia (14%), and diarrhea (13%); the incidence of febrile neutropenia was 7%. IMMU-132 was well-tolerated and showed promising activity in heavily pretreated patients with metastatic TNBC. Preclinical studies combining IMMU-132 with PARP inhibitors and taxanes have shown synthetic lethality, and further investigation is underway [79, 80].

9.11.2 Glembatumumab Vedotin

Glycoprotein nonmetastatic B (gpNMB), a type I transmembrane protein, is overexpressed in 40–60% of breast cancers [81, 82]. Associated with the basal-like subtype and poor prognosis, overexpression of gpNMB promotes invasion and metastasis, decreases tumor cell apoptosis, and promotes angiogenesis in preclinical models [81, 83]. Glembatumumab vedotin (CDX-011; formerly CR011-vcMMAE) is an ADC consisting of CDX-011, a fully human IgG2 monoclonal antibody against gpNMB, and monomethyl auristatin E (MMAE), a potent microtubule inhibitor [84, 85]. Glembatumumab vedotin is designed to bind to gpNMB and, after internalization, release MMAE via cleavage of a protease-sensitive valine-citrulline peptide linker, resulting in tumor cell death by microtubule inhibition [86].

In a phase I/II clinical trial of heavily pretreated patients (median of seven prior regimens) with advanced breast cancer, glembatumumab vedotin, dosed at 1.88 mg/kg intravenously every 3 weeks, had an acceptable safety profile with an ORR 12% (4 of 33 patients) and median PFS of 9.1 weeks [87]. The primary efficacy endpoint for the phase II portion of the study was met (12-week progression-free survival [PFS12] = 9 of 27 patients; 33%). Fatigue, rash, nausea, peripheral sensory neuropathy, and neutropenia were the most frequent treatment-related AEs. In TNBC patients, ORR was 20% (2 of 10) and median PFS was 17.9 weeks, and in the subset of TNBC patients with gpNMB-expressing tumors (≥5% of epithelial or stromal cells positive), ORR was 25% (1 of 4), and median PFS was 5.1 months.

Based on these results, the open-label, randomized, phase II EMERGE study was initiated to evaluate the activity of glembatumumab vedotin in advanced gpNMB-expressing breast cancer (CDX011-03; A Study of Glembatumumab Vedotin in Patients with Advanced GPNMB-expressing Breast Cancer) [88]. In the study, 124 patients with refractory breast cancer expressing gpNMB in ≥5% of epithelial or stromal cells were randomized to receive glembatumumab vedotin (n = 83) or investigator's choice of chemotherapy (IC) (n = 41). Patients had received a median of four lines of prior systemic therapy for advanced or metastatic disease. The primary endpoint was to detect an ORR in the glembatumumab vedotin group between 10 and 22.5%. The study did not meet its primary endpoint, with an ORR of 6% in the glembatumumab vedotin group vs. 7% in the IC group, and no evidence of between-group difference in ORR in the three defined strata (gpNMB expression in tumor epithelial cells or low vs. high intensity in stromal cells). However, the response rates among patients with gpNMB expression in ≥25% of tumor epithelial cells were 30% (7/23) in the glembatumumab vedotin group vs. 9% (1/11) in the IC group. Further, unplanned analysis showed response rates of 18% (5/28) vs. 0% (0/11) in patients with TNBC and 40% (4/10) vs. 0% (0/6) in the small subset of patients with gpNMB-overexpressing triple-negative disease. The most common TRAEs were rash, neutropenia, peripheral neuropathy, alopecia, and pruritus. The investigators concluded that although the primary endpoint in advanced gpNMB-expressing breast cancer was not met for all enrolled patients, activity may be enhanced in patients with gpNMB-overexpressing tumors and/or TNBC. The Metastatic Triple-Negative Breast Cancer (METRIC) study is an international, randomized phase II trial comparing glembatumumab vedotin to capecitabine in patients with metastatic gpNMB-over-expressing TNBC (NCT00071942) [89].

9.11.3 SGN-LIV1A

LIV-1 is a multi-span transmembrane protein with zinc transporter and metallopro-teinase activity that is upregulated in TNBC [90–92]. By interacting with the tran-scription factors STAT3 and Snail to downregulate expression of E-cadherin and promote epithelial-mesenchymal transition (EMT), LIV-1 expression has been linked to malignant progression and metastasis [93–96]. SGN-LIV1A is an antibody-drug conjugate made from a humanized anti-LIV-1 antibody (hLIV22) conjugated through a proteolytically cleavable linker to monomethyl auristatin E (MMAE), a potent microtubule inhibitor. Upon binding to cell surface LIV-1, SGN-LIV1A is internalized and releases MMAE, which binds to tubulin and induces G2/M arrest and apoptosis [84, 92].

In a phase I dose-escalation study evaluating SGN-LIV1A in heavily pre-treated women with advanced or metastatic breast cancer, 39 patients (21 TNBC, 18 HR+/HER2-negative) have received a median of three cycles (range, 1–10) of SGN-LIV1A monotherapy at doses of 0.5–2.8 mg/kg intravenously every 3 weeks [97]. Among the 17 efficacy evaluable (EE) TNBC patients, the objective response rate (ORR = CR + PR) was 41% (7 PR), the disease control rate (DCR = CR + PR + SD) was 82% (7 PR, 7 SD), and the clinical benefit rate (CBR = ORR + SD ≥24 weeks) was 53% (nine patients). For TNBC patients, median PFS was 17.1 weeks (95% CI, 6.0–18.4 weeks). Of 281 metastatic breast cancer tumor samples evaluated for LIV-1 expression, 93% were positive; 81% had moderate-to-high expression (H-score ≥ 100). No DLTs occurred in 19 DLT-evaluable patients, and the maximum tolerated dose was not exceeded at 2.8 mg/kg. The most common treatment-related AEs reported in ≥30% of patients were fatigue, nausea, alopecia, decreased appetite, constipation, neutropenia, and vomiting. Peripheral neuropathy was reported in nine patients (23%). Response duration data continue to evolve, and enrollment continues in the TNBC mono-therapy expansion cohort.

Conclusion

TNBC is a molecularly diverse and heterogeneous disease. The identification of several specific subtypes of TNBC is key to the delivery of more personalized treatments for TNBC. Ongoing clinical trials and future clinical research in the different subgroups of TNBC will help to validate the efficacy of such novel treatment strategies.

References

1. Perou CM, Sorlie T, Eisen MB, van de Rijn M, Jeffrey SS, Rees CA, et al. Molecular portraits of human breast tumours. Nature. 2000;406(6797):747–52.
2. Sorlie T, Perou CM, Tibshirani R, Aas T, Geisler S, Johnsen H, et al. Gene expression patterns of breast carcinomas distinguish tumor subclasses with clinical implications. Proc Natl Acad Sci U S A. 2001;98(19):10869–74.
3. Lehmann BD, Bauer JA, Chen X, Sanders ME, Chakravarthy AB, Shyr Y, et al. Identification of human triple-negative breast cancer subtypes and preclinical models for selection of targeted therapies. J Clin Invest. 2011;121(7):2750–67.
4. Lehmann BD, Jovanovic B, Chen X, Estrada MV, Johnson KN, Shyr Y, et al. Refinement of triple-negative breast cancer molecular subtypes: implications for neoadjuvant chemotherapy selection. PLoS One. 2016;11(6):e0157368.
5. Cancer Genome Atlas N. Comprehensive molecular portraits of human breast tumours. Nature. 2012;490(7418):61–70.
6. Parker JS, Mullins M, Cheang MC, Leung S, Voduc D, Vickery T, et al. Supervised risk predictor of breast cancer based on intrinsic subtypes. J Clin Oncol. 2009;27(8):1160–7.
7. Rahim F, Hajizamani S, Mortaz E, Ahmadzadeh A, Shahjahani M, Shahrabi S, et al. Molecular regulation of bone marrow metastasis in prostate and breast cancer. Bone marrow Res. 2014;2014:405920.
8. Masuda H, Baggerly KA, Wang Y, Zhang Y, Gonzalez-Angulo AM, Meric-Bernstam F, et al. Differential response to neoadjuvant chemotherapy among 7 triple-negative breast cancer molecular subtypes. Clin Cancer Res. 2013;19(19):5533–40.
9. Burstein MD, Tsimelzon A, Poage GM, Covington KR, Contreras A, Fuqua SA, et al. Comprehensive genomic analysis identifies novel subtypes and targets of triple-negative breast cancer. Clin Cancer Res. 2015;21(7):1688–98.
10. Tutt A, Ashworth A. The relationship between the roles of BRCA genes in DNA repair and cancer predisposition. Trends Mol Med. 2002;8(12):571–6.
11. Venkitaraman AR. Cancer susceptibility and the functions of BRCA1 and BRCA2. Cell. 2002;108(2):171–82.
12. Donawho CK, Luo Y, Luo Y, Penning TD, Bauch JL, Bouska JJ, et al. ABT-888, an orally active poly(ADP-ribose) polymerase inhibitor that potentiates DNA-damaging agents in preclinical tumor models. Clin Cancer Res. 2007;13(9):2728–37.
13. Pommier Y, O'Connor MJ, de Bono J. Laying a trap to kill cancer cells: PARP inhibitors and their mechanisms of action. Sci Transl Med. 2016;8(362):362ps17.
14. Farmer H, McCabe N, Lord CJ, Tutt AN, Johnson DA, Richardson TB, et al. Targeting the DNA repair defect in BRCA mutant cells as a therapeutic strategy. Nature. 2005;434(7035):917–21.
15. Kaelin WG Jr. The concept of synthetic lethality in the context of anticancer therapy. Nat Rev Cancer. 2005;5(9):689–98.
16. Fong PC, Boss DS, Yap TA, Tutt A, Wu P, Mergui-Roelvink M, et al. Inhibition of poly(ADP-ribose) polymerase in tumors from BRCA mutation carriers. N Engl J Med. 2009;361(2):123–34.
17. Tutt A, Robson M, Garber JE, Domchek SM, Audeh MW, Weitzel JN, et al. Oral poly(ADP-ribose) polymerase inhibitor olaparib in patients with BRCA1 or BRCA2 mutations and advanced breast cancer: a proof-of-concept trial. Lancet (Lond Engl). 2010;376(9737):235–44.
18. Kaufman B, Shapira-Frommer R, Schmutzler RK, Audeh MW, Friedlander M, Balmana J, et al. Olaparib monotherapy in patients with advanced cancer and a germline BRCA1/2 mutation. J Clin Oncol. 2015;33(3):244–50.
19. Robson M, Im SA, Senkus E, Xu B, Domchek SM, Masuda N, et al. Olaparib for metastatic breast cancer in patients with a germline BRCA mutation. N Engl J Med. 2017.

20. Tutt ANJ, Kaufman B, Gelber RD, Fadden EM, Goessl CD, Viale G, et al. OlympiA: a randomized phase III trial of olaparib as adjuvant therapy in patients with high-risk HER2-negative breast cancer (BC) and a germline BRCA1/2 mutation (gBRCAm). J Clin Oncol. 2015;33(15_suppl):TPS1109-TPS.
21. Isakoff SJ, Overmoyer B, Tung NM, Gelman RS, Giranda VL, Bernhard KM, et al. A phase II trial of the PARP inhibitor veliparib (ABT888) and temozolomide for metastatic breast cancer. J Clin Oncol. 2010;28(15_suppl):1019.
22. Somlo G, Frankel PH, Arun BK, Ma CX, Garcia AA, Cigler T, et al. Efficacy of the PARP inhibitor veliparib with carboplatin or as a single agent in patients with germline BRCA1- or BRCA2-associated metastatic breast cancer: California Cancer Consortium Trial NCT01149083. Clin Cancer Res. 2017.
23. Isakoff S, Overmoyer B, Tung N, Gelman R, Habin K, Qian J, et al. P3-16-05: a phase II trial expansion cohort of the PARP inhibitor veliparib (ABT888) and temozolomide in BRCA1/2 associated metastatic breast cancer. Cancer Res. 2011;71(24 Supplement):P3-16-05-P3-16-05.
24. Isakoff SJ, Puhalla S, Domchek SM, Friedlander M, Kaufman B, Robson M, et al. A randomized phase II study of veliparib with temozolomide or carboplatin/paclitaxel versus placebo with carboplatin/paclitaxel in BRCA1/2 metastatic breast cancer: design and rationale. Future Oncol (Lond Engl). 2017;13(4):307–20.
25. Diéras V, Han H, Robson M, Palácová M, Marcom P, Jager A, et al. Abstract P4-22-02: evaluation of veliparib (V) and temozolomide (TMZ) in a phase 2 randomized study of the efficacy and tolerability of V+TMZ or carboplatin (C) and paclitaxel (P) vs placebo (Plc)+C/P in patients (pts) with BRCA1 or BRCA2 mutations and metastatic breast cancer. Cancer Res. 2017;77(4 Supplement):P4-22-02-P4-22-02.
26. Han H, Diéras V, Robson M, Palácová M, Marcom P, Jager A, et al. Abstract S2-05: efficacy and tolerability of veliparib (V; ABT-888) in combination with carboplatin (C) and paclitaxel (P) vs placebo (Plc)+C/P in patients (pts) with BRCA1 or BRCA2 mutations and metastatic breast cancer: a randomized, phase 2 study. Cancer Res. 2017;77(4 Suppl):S2-05-S2-05.
27. Balmana J, Tryfonidis K, Audeh W, Goulioti T, Slaets L, Agarwal S, et al. Abstract OT1-03-05: a phase III, randomized, open label, multicenter, controlled trial of niraparib versus physician's choice in previously treated, HER2 negative, germline BRCA mutation-positive breast cancer patients. An EORTC-BIG intergroup study (BRAVO study). Cancer Res. 2016;76(4 Suppl):OT1-03-5-OT1-03-5.
28. Litton J, Ettl J, Hurvitz S, Mina L, Rugo H, Lee K-H, et al. Abstract OT2-01-13: a phase 3, open-label, randomized, 2-arm international study of the oral dual PARP inhibitor talazoparib in germline BRCA mutation subjects with locally advanced and/or metastatic breast cancer (EMBRACA). Cancer Res. 2017;77(4 Supplement):OT2-01-13-OT2-01-13.
29. Hartman AR, Kaldate RR, Sailer LM, Painter L, Grier CE, Endsley RR, et al. Prevalence of BRCA mutations in an unselected population of triple-negative breast cancer. Cancer. 2012;118(11):2787–95.
30. Turner N, Tutt A, Ashworth A. Hallmarks of 'BRCAness' in sporadic cancers. Nat Rev Cancer. 2004;4(10):814–9.
31. Lord CJ, Ashworth A. BRCAness revisited. Nat Rev Cancer. 2016;16(2):110–20.
32. Rugo HS, Olopade OI, DeMichele A, Yau C, van't Veer LJ, Buxton MB, et al. Adaptive randomization of veliparib-carboplatin treatment in breast cancer. N Engl J Med. 2016;375(1):23–34.
33. Geyer CE, O'Shaughnessy J, Untch M, Sikov W, Rugo HS, McKee MD, et al. Phase 3 study evaluating efficacy and safety of veliparib (V) plus carboplatin (Cb) or Cb in combination with standard neoadjuvant chemotherapy (NAC) in patients (pts) with early stage triple-negative breast cancer (TNBC). J Clin Oncol. 2017;35(15_suppl):520.
34. Barton VN, D'Amato NC, Gordon MA, Lind HT, Spoelstra NS, Babbs BL, et al. Multiple molecular subtypes of triple-negative breast cancer critically rely on androgen receptor and respond to enzalutamide in vivo. Mol Cancer Ther. 2015;14(3):769–78.
35. Loibl S, Muller BM, von Minckwitz G, Schwabe M, Roller M, Darb-Esfahani S, et al. Androgen receptor expression in primary breast cancer and its predictive and prognostic value in patients treated with neoadjuvant chemotherapy. Breast Cancer Res Treat. 2011;130(2):477–87.

36. Gucalp A, Tolaney S, Isakoff SJ, Ingle JN, Liu MC, Carey LA, et al. Phase II trial of bicalutamide in patients with androgen receptor-positive, estrogen receptor-negative metastatic breast cancer. Clin Cancer Res. 2013;19(19):5505–12.
37. Hammond ME, Hayes DF, Dowsett M, Allred DC, Hagerty KL, Badve S, et al. American Society of Clinical Oncology/College of American Pathologists guideline recommendations for immunohistochemical testing of estrogen and progesterone receptors in breast cancer. J Clin Oncol. 2010;28(16):2784–95.
38. Bonnefoi H, Grellety T, Tredan O, Saghatchian M, Dalenc F, Mailliez A, et al. A phase II trial of abiraterone acetate plus prednisone in patients with triple-negative androgen receptor positive locally advanced or metastatic breast cancer (UCBG 12-1). Ann Oncol. 2016;27(5):812–8.
39. Traina TA, Miller K, Yardley DA, O'Shaughnessy J, Cortes J, Awada A, et al. Results from a phase 2 study of enzalutamide (ENZA), an androgen receptor (AR) inhibitor, in advanced AR+ triple-negative breast cancer (TNBC). J Clin Oncol. 2015;33(15_suppl):1003.
40. Parker JS, Peterson AC, Tudor IC, Hoffman J, Uppal H. A novel biomarker to predict sensitivity to enzalutamide (ENZA) in TNBC. J Clin Oncol. 2015;33(15_suppl):1083.
41. Traina TA, Yardley DA, Schwartzberg LS, O'Shaughnessy J, Cortes J, Awada A, et al. Overall survival (OS) in patients (Pts) with diagnostic positive (Dx+) breast cancer: subgroup analysis from a phase 2 study of enzalutamide (ENZA), an androgen receptor (AR) inhibitor, in AR+ triple-negative breast cancer (TNBC) treated with 0-1 prior lines of therapy. J Clin Oncol. 2017;35(15_suppl):1089.
42. Conzen SD. Minireview: nuclear receptors and breast cancer. Mol Endocrinol (Baltimore, MD). 2008;22(10):2215–28.
43. Mikosz CA, Brickley DR, Sharkey MS, Moran TW, Conzen SD. Glucocorticoid receptor-mediated protection from apoptosis is associated with induction of the serine/threonine survival kinase gene, sgk-1. J Biol Chem. 2001;276(20):16649–54.
44. Skor MN, Wonder EL, Kocherginsky M, Goyal A, Hall BA, Cai Y, et al. Glucocorticoid receptor antagonism as a novel therapy for triple-negative breast cancer. Clin Cancer Res. 2013;19(22):6163–72.
45. Pan D, Kocherginsky M, Conzen SD. Activation of the glucocorticoid receptor is associated with poor prognosis in estrogen receptor-negative breast cancer. Cancer Res. 2011;71(20):6360–70.
46. Nanda R, Stringer-Reasor EM, Saha P, Kocherginsky M, Gibson J, Libao B, et al. A randomized phase I trial of nanoparticle albumin-bound paclitaxel with or without mifepristone for advanced breast cancer. SpringerPlus. 2016;5(1):947.
47. Stringer EM, Saha P, Swoboda A, Kocherginsky M, Baker G, Olberkyte S, et al. A phase I trial of mifepristone (M), carboplatin (C), and gemcitabine (G) in advanced breast and ovarian cancer. J Clin Oncol. 2017;35(15_suppl):1083.
48. Freeman GJ, Long AJ, Iwai Y, Bourque K, Chernova T, Nishimura H, et al. Engagement of the PD-1 immunoinhibitory receptor by a novel B7 family member leads to negative regulation of lymphocyte activation. J Exp Med. 2000;192(7):1027–34.
49. Latchman Y, Wood CR, Chernova T, Chaudhary D, Borde M, Chernova I, et al. PD-L2 is a second ligand for PD-1 and inhibits T cell activation. Nat Immunol. 2001;2(3):261–8.
50. Francisco LM, Salinas VH, Brown KE, Vanguri VK, Freeman GJ, Kuchroo VK, et al. PD-L1 regulates the development, maintenance, and function of induced regulatory T cells. J Exp Med. 2009;206(13):3015–29.
51. Amarnath S, Mangus CW, Wang JC, Wei F, He A, Kapoor V, et al. The PDL1-PD1 axis converts human TH1 cells into regulatory T cells. Sci Transl Med. 2011;3(111):111ra20.
52. Spranger S, Spaapen RM, Zha Y, Williams J, Meng Y, Ha TT, et al. Up-regulation of PD-L1, IDO, and T(regs) in the melanoma tumor microenvironment is driven by CD8(+) T cells. Sci Transl Med. 2013;5(200):200ra116.
53. Kinter AL, Godbout EJ, McNally JP, Sereti I, Roby GA, O'Shea MA, et al. The common gamma-chain cytokines IL-2, IL-7, IL-15, and IL-21 induce the expression of programmed death-1 and its ligands. J Immunol. 2008;181(10):6738–46.

54. Nanda R, Chow LQ, Dees EC, Berger R, Gupta S, Geva R, et al. Pembrolizumab in patients with advanced triple-negative breast cancer: phase Ib KEYNOTE-012 study. J Clin Oncol. 2016;34(21):2460–7.
55. Adams S, Schmid P, Rugo HS, Winer EP, Loirat D, Awada A, et al. Phase 2 study of pembrolizumab (pembro) monotherapy for previously treated metastatic triple-negative breast cancer (mTNBC): KEYNOTE-086 cohort A. J Clin Oncol. 2017;35(15_suppl):1008.
56. Adams S, Loi S, Toppmeyer D, Cescon DW, Laurentiis MD, Nanda R, et al. Phase 2 study of pembrolizumab as first-line therapy for PD-L1–positive metastatic triple-negative breast cancer (mTNBC): preliminary data from KEYNOTE-086 cohort B. J Clin Oncol. 2017;35(15_suppl):1088.
57. Winer EP, Dang T, Karantza V, Su S-C. KEYNOTE-119: a randomized phase III study of single-agent pembrolizumab (MK-3475) vs single-agent chemotherapy per physician's choice for metastatic triple-negative breast cancer (mTNBC). J Clin Oncol. 2016;34(15_suppl):TPS1102-TPS.
58. Tolaney S, Savulsky C, Aktan G, Xing D, Almonte A, Karantza V, et al. Abstract P5-15-02: phase 1b/2 study to evaluate eribulin mesylate in combination with pembrolizumab in patients with metastatic triple-negative breast cancer. Cancer Res. 2017;77(4 Suppl):P5-15-02-P5-15-02.
59. Nanda R, Liu MC, Yau C, Asare S, Hylton N, Veer LV, et al. Pembrolizumab plus standard neoadjuvant therapy for high-risk breast cancer (BC): results from I-SPY 2. J Clin Oncol. 2017;35(15_suppl):506.
60. Herbst RS, Soria JC, Kowanetz M, Fine GD, Hamid O, Gordon MS, et al. Predictive correlates of response to the anti-PD-L1 antibody MPDL3280A in cancer patients. Nature. 2014;515(7528):563–7.
61. Powles T, Eder JP, Fine GD, Braiteh FS, Loriot Y, Cruz C, et al. MPDL3280A (anti-PD-L1) treatment leads to clinical activity in metastatic bladder cancer. Nature. 2014;515(7528):558–62.
62. Emens LA, Braiteh FS, Cassier P, Delord J-P, Eder JP, Fasso M, et al. Abstract 2859: inhibition of PD-L1 by MPDL3280A leads to clinical activity in patients with metastatic triple-negative breast cancer (TNBC). Cancer Res. 2015;75(15 Suppl):2859.
63. Hodi FS, Hwu WJ, Kefford R, Weber JS, Daud A, Hamid O, et al. Evaluation of immune-related response criteria and RECIST v1.1 in patients with advanced melanoma treated with pembrolizumab. J Clin Oncol. 2016;34(13):1510–7.
64. Adams S, Diamond JR, Hamilton EP, Pohlmann PR, Tolaney SM, Molinero L, et al. Phase Ib trial of atezolizumab in combination with nab-paclitaxel in patients with metastatic triple-negative breast cancer (mTNBC). J Clin Oncol. 2016;34(15_suppl):1009.
65. Emens LA, Adams S, Loi S, Schneeweiss A, Rugo HS, Winer EP, et al. IMpassion130: a phase III randomized trial of atezolizumab with nab-paclitaxel for first-line treatment of patients with metastatic triple-negative breast cancer (mTNBC). J Clin Oncol. 2016;34(15_suppl):TPS1104-TPS.
66. Dirix L, Takacs I, Nikolinakos P, Jerusalem G, Arkenau H-T, Hamilton E, et al. Abstract S1-04: Avelumab (MSB0010718C), an anti-PD-L1 antibody, in patients with locally advanced or metastatic breast cancer: a phase Ib JAVELIN solid tumor trial. Cancer Res. 2016;76(4 Suppl):S1-04-S1.
67. Cantley LC. The phosphoinositide 3-kinase pathway. Science (New York, NY). 2002;296(5573):1655–7.
68. Manning BD, Cantley LC. AKT/PKB signaling: navigating downstream. Cell. 2007;129(7):1261–74.
69. Bhaskar PT, Hay N. The two TORCs and Akt. Dev Cell. 2007;12(4):487–502.
70. Tripathy D, Chien AJ, Hylton N, Buxton MB, Ewing CA, Wallace AM, et al. Adaptively randomized trial of neoadjuvant chemotherapy with or without the Akt inhibitor MK-2206: graduation results from the I-SPY 2 trial. J Clin Oncol. 2015;33(15_suppl):524.
71. Kim SB, Dent R, Im SA, Espie M, Blau S, Tan AR, et al. Ipatasertib plus paclitaxel versus placebo plus paclitaxel as first-line therapy for metastatic triple-negative breast cancer (LOTUS): a multicentre, randomised, double-blind, placebo-controlled, phase 2 trial. Lancet Oncol. 2017;18(10):1360–72.

72. Ambrogi F, Fornili M, Boracchi P, Trerotola M, Relli V, Simeone P, et al. Trop-2 is a determinant of breast cancer survival. PLoS One. 2014;9(5):e96993.
73. Starodub AN, Ocean AJ, Shah MA, Guarino MJ, Picozzi VJ Jr, Vahdat LT, et al. First-in-human trial of a novel anti-trop-2 antibody-SN-38 conjugate, sacituzumab govitecan, for the treatment of diverse metastatic solid tumors. Clin Cancer Res. 2015;21(17):3870–8.
74. Sharkey RM, McBride WJ, Cardillo TM, Govindan SV, Wang Y, Rossi EA, et al. Enhanced delivery of SN-38 to human tumor xenografts with an anti-trop-2-SN-38 antibody conjugate (sacituzumab govitecan). Clin Cancer Res. 2015;21(22):5131–8.
75. Goldenberg DM, Cardillo TM, Govindan SV, Rossi EA, Sharkey RM. Trop-2 is a novel target for solid cancer therapy with sacituzumab govitecan (IMMU-132), an antibody-drug conjugate (ADC). Oncotarget. 2015;6(26):22496–512.
76. Cardillo TM, Govindan SV, Sharkey RM, Trisal P, Arrojo R, Liu D, et al. Sacituzumab govitecan (IMMU-132), an anti-trop-2/SN-38 antibody-drug conjugate: characterization and efficacy in pancreatic, gastric, and other cancers. Bioconjug Chem. 2015;26(5):919–31.
77. Rothenberg ML. Topoisomerase I inhibitors: review and update. Ann Oncol. 1997;8(9):837–55.
78. Bardia A, Mayer IA, Diamond JR, Moroose RL, Isakoff SJ, Starodub AN, et al. Efficacy and safety of anti-trop-2 antibody drug conjugate sacituzumab govitecan (IMMU-132) in heavily pretreated patients with metastatic triple-negative breast cancer. J Clin Oncol. 2017;35(19):2141–8.
79. Goldenberg D, Cardillo T, Govindan S, Zalath M, Arrojo R, Sharkey R. Abstract P6-15-02: synthetic lethality in TNBC mediated by an anti-Trop-2 antibody-drug conjugate, sacituzumab govitecan (IMMU-132), when combined with paclitaxel or the PARP inhibitor, olaparib. Cancer Res. 2016;76(4 Suppl):P6-15-02-P6-15-02.
80. Cardillo TM, Sharkey RM, Rossi DL, Arrojo R, Mostafa AA, Goldenberg DM. Synthetic lethality exploitation by an anti-trop-2-SN-38 antibody-drug conjugate, IMMU-132, plus PARP inhibitors in BRCA1/2-wild-type triple-negative breast cancer. Clin Cancer Res. 2017;23(13):3405–15.
81. Rose AA, Grosset AA, Dong Z, Russo C, Macdonald PA, Bertos NR, et al. Glycoprotein nonmetastatic B is an independent prognostic indicator of recurrence and a novel therapeutic target in breast cancer. Clin Cancer Res. 2010;16(7):2147–56.
82. Ripoll VM, Irvine KM, Ravasi T, Sweet MJ, Hume DA. Gpnmb is induced in macrophages by IFN-gamma and lipopolysaccharide and acts as a feedback regulator of proinflammatory responses. J Immunol. 2007;178(10):6557–66.
83. Rose AA, Pepin F, Russo C, Abou Khalil JE, Hallett M, Siegel PM. Osteoactivin promotes breast cancer metastasis to bone. Mol Cancer Res. 2007;5(10):1001–14.
84. Doronina SO, Toki BE, Torgov MY, Mendelsohn BA, Cerveny CG, Chace DF, et al. Development of potent monoclonal antibody auristatin conjugates for cancer therapy. Nat Biotechnol. 2003;21(7):778–84.
85. Naumovski L, Junutula JR. Glembatumumab vedotin, a conjugate of an anti-glycoprotein non-metastatic melanoma protein B mAb and monomethyl auristatin E for the treatment of melanoma and breast cancer. Curr Opin Mol Ther. 2010;12(2):248–57.
86. Sutherland MS, Sanderson RJ, Gordon KA, Andreyka J, Cerveny CG, Yu C, et al. Lysosomal trafficking and cysteine protease metabolism confer target-specific cytotoxicity by peptide-linked anti-CD30-auristatin conjugates. J Biol Chem. 2006;281(15):10540–7.
87. Bendell J, Saleh M, Rose AA, Siegel PM, Hart L, Sirpal S, et al. Phase I/II study of the antibody-drug conjugate glembatumumab vedotin in patients with locally advanced or metastatic breast cancer. J Clin Oncol. 2014;32(32):3619–25.
88. Yardley DA, Weaver R, Melisko ME, Saleh MN, Arena FP, Forero A, et al. EMERGE: a randomized phase II study of the antibody-drug conjugate glembatumumab vedotin in advanced glycoprotein NMB-expressing breast cancer. J Clin Oncol. 2015;33(14):1609–19.
89. Schmid P, Melisko M, Yardley DA, Blackwell K, Forero A, Ouellette G, et al. METRIC: a randomized international study of the antibody drug conjugate (ADC) glembatumumab vedotin (GV, CDX-011) in patients (pts) with metastatic gpNMB overexpressing triple-negative breast cancer (TNBC). Ann Oncol. 2016;27(suppl_6):309TiP-TiP.

90. Taylor KM, Morgan HE, Johnson A, Hadley LJ, Nicholson RI. Structure-function analysis of LIV-1, the breast cancer-associated protein that belongs to a new subfamily of zinc transporters. Biochem J. 2003;375(Pt 1):51–9.
91. Lopez V, Kelleher SL. Zip6-attenuation promotes epithelial-to-mesenchymal transition in ductal breast tumor (T47D) cells. Exp Cell Res. 2010;316(3):366–75.
92. Sussman D, Smith LM, Anderson ME, Duniho S, Hunter JH, Kostner H, et al. SGN-LIV1A: a novel antibody-drug conjugate targeting LIV-1 for the treatment of metastatic breast cancer. Mol Cancer Ther. 2014;13(12):2991–3000.
93. Huber MA, Kraut N, Beug H. Molecular requirements for epithelial-mesenchymal transition during tumor progression. Curr Opin Cell Biol. 2005;17(5):548–58.
94. Taylor KM, Hiscox S, Nicholson RI. Zinc transporter LIV-1: a link between cellular development and cancer progression. Trends Endocrinol Metab. 2004;15(10):461–3.
95. Unno J, Satoh K, Hirota M, Kanno A, Hamada S, Ito H, et al. LIV-1 enhances the aggressive phenotype through the induction of epithelial to mesenchymal transition in human pancreatic carcinoma cells. Int J Oncol. 2009;35(4):813–21.
96. Lue HW, Yang X, Wang R, Qian W, RZ X, Lyles R, et al. LIV-1 promotes prostate cancer epithelial-to-mesenchymal transition and metastasis through HB-EGF shedding and EGFR-mediated ERK signaling. PLoS One. 2011;6(11):e27720.
97. Forero-Torres A, Modi S, Specht J, Miller K, Weise A, Burris H, et al. Abstract P6-12-04: phase 1 study of the antibody-drug conjugate (ADC) SGN-LIV1A in patients with heavily pretreated metastatic breast cancer. Cancer Res. 2017;77(4 Suppl):P6-12-04-P6-12-04.

Special Issues in Young Women with Triple-Negative Breast Cancer

10

Narjust Duma, Ciara C. O'Sullivan, Kathryn J. Ruddy, and Alexis D. Leal

Clinical Pearls
- Though young patients with triple-negative breast cancer are usually treated aggressively due to poorer prognosis and few competing health concerns, treatment recommendations should be based on stage and biological characteristics of the tumor and not based on young age alone.
- Discussion of fertility preservation and/or referral to a reproductive specialist to discuss fertility preservation options prior to chemotherapy is recommended in a young patient with triple-negative breast cancer.
- Unique considerations for young women with triple-negative breast cancer are premature menopause with subsequent sexual dysfunction, reduced fertility, increased social stressors from raising young children and navigating active workforce participation, and a prolonged survivorship period.

10.1 Introduction

Triple-negative breast cancer (TNBC) is more frequently seen in younger women [1]. The cutoff age for a "young breast cancer patient" ranges from 35 to 50 years across the literature, so we will focus on the unique challenges experienced by women who are 50 years of age or younger at diagnosis. In the United States,

N. Duma, MD • C.C. O'Sullivan, MB, BCh • K.J. Ruddy, MD, MPH (✉)
Department of Oncology, Mayo Clinic College of Medicine and Science,
Mayo Clinic, Rochester, MN, USA
e-mail: duma.narjust@mayo.edu; osullivan.ciara@mayo.edu
ruddy.kathryn@mayo.edu

A.D. Leal, MD
Division of Medical Oncology, University of Colorado Cancer Center, Aurora, CO, USA
e-mail: alexis.leal@ucdenver.edu

© Springer International Publishing AG 2018
A.R. Tan (ed.), *Triple-Negative Breast Cancer*,
https://doi.org/10.1007/978-3-319-69980-6_10

approximately 46,000 women <50 years are diagnosed with breast cancer each year [2]. Young women tend to present with more aggressive, advanced disease at diagnosis and have a higher risk of dying from their disease than older women [3–6]. In this chapter, we will address tumor biology, delays in diagnosis, genetic testing, treatment considerations and related toxicities, psychosocial issues, healthcare disparities, sexual functioning, fertility preservation, contraception, future childbearing, and quality of life (QOL) issues.

10.1.1 Delayed Diagnosis

Greater than 90% of young women with breast cancer are symptomatic at diagnosis, with large tumors and nodal involvement [7, 8]. Young women may be more prone to experience delays in diagnosis than their older counterparts because neither the patient nor the physician strongly suspects the diagnosis [9, 10]. In addition, for those who do have breast imaging either to screen for or work up a breast abnormality, the high breast density in many young women makes interpretation of breast imaging difficult [11]. Physiological changes during pregnancy and lactation can also contribute to diagnostic difficulties. In one retrospective study, 239 women diagnosed with breast cancer under age 40 were compared with 2101 women aged ≥40 at the time of a breast cancer diagnosis [7]. On mammography, lesions in younger women were more likely to be undetected or interpreted as benign, particularly in women with dense breasts. An abnormality was detected on ultrasound in 92.2% of cancers in young women but was more likely to have been considered benign than in older women. However, the data about delays in the diagnosis of breast cancer in young women have been mixed. In one prospective multicenter study of 585 women (aged ≤40) with recently diagnosed breast cancer, delays of at least 90 days were assessed, both between the first sign or symptom and seeking medical attention (defined as "self-delay") and between seeking medical attention and receiving a diagnosis of breast cancer (defined as "care delay"). In this study, only 17% reported self-delay, and only 12% reported care delay. The median time between the initial sign and seeking medical attention was only 14 days, and the median time between seeking medical attention and diagnosis was 16.5 days [12].

10.1.2 Pathology and Biology of Triple-Negative Breast Cancer in Young Women

Several studies have attempted to elucidate biological differences that might drive poorer TNBC prognoses in young women [13–16]. Some detected differences in gene expression, but did not control for the effect of different subtypes of breast cancer [17]. Results from subsequent studies that included tumor subtype and clinical features inferred that age alone may not provide further complexity among breast cancer subtypes [1].

10.1.3 Genetic Testing

Up to 40% of women diagnosed before 40 years of age with TNBC have a deleterious germline *BRCA* mutation (*gBRCAm*). Therefore, referral to a cancer genetics professional to discuss genetic testing should be considered at diagnosis for all women with TNBC ≤60 years [18], as results could impact treatment decisions and may have far-reaching implications for other family members. There is a strong association between *gBRCA1m* and TNBC, with 60–80% of tumors that develop in these patients having this phenotype, and the association is strongest in women aged <50 [19]. Further, *gBRCA1m* are present in approximately 29% of women diagnosed with TNBC who have Ashkenazi Jewish ancestry [20]. These women are at high risk for the development of contralateral breast cancer, with an estimated cumulative risk of 20–83% among those who harbor a deleterious mutation [21–23]. Some women who have a *gBRCA1/2m* may be more inclined to pursue a contralateral prophylactic mastectomy to reduce their future cancer risk. However, this varies internationally [24]. Interestingly, one study investigating the incidence of *BRCA* mutations among patients with TNBC and the prognostic implications of these mutations found that the risk of relapse in patients with TNBC and a *gBRCA1m* was significantly decreased when compared to those who did not harbor a mutation [25].

10.2 General Treatment Considerations

10.2.1 Surgery

Despite widespread acceptance of breast-conserving surgery (BCS), there was initial reluctance to apply these findings to young women due to their higher risk of local recurrence. Although the initial randomized trials that established the efficacy of BCS included women of all ages, young women represented a relatively small proportion of patients, which may contribute to the lower BCS rates in this subgroup. A recent patterns-of-care analysis revealed that young women have a higher mastectomy rate, and this has significantly increased over the past decade [26]. Bilateral mastectomies are particularly popular in younger women [27–29]. Desire for breast symmetry plays a role in this decision for some women [30]. Furthermore, women with breast cancer may overestimate their risks of future breast cancer events [31]. In a cross-sectional study of 123 women ≤40 years who underwent contralateral prophylactic mastectomy, the vast majority (>90%) indicated that their motivation was to reduce the risk of contralateral breast cancer and improve survival [32], a finding which has been reproduced in other studies [32–34]. This mismatch between perceived and actual risk should be addressed with careful counseling and education. Although it is important for providers to respect the rationale behind patient decision-making in this setting, surgical complications and long-term sequelae also need to be considered. After more extensive surgery, women are more likely to experience postoperative chest numbness or chronic pain that may be long-lasting and may significantly impact quality of life. The benefits of BCS often include superior cosmetic outcomes and a faster recovery, allowing young patients an earlier return to "normal life" (work, caring for children or elderly parents, etc.). Further, some studies suggest that BCS may abrogate the feelings of loss of femininity commonly associated with breast cancer treatment [35].

10.2.2 Radiotherapy

Radiotherapy is often an important component in the management of young women with stage I to III TNBC, improving local control and survival outcomes [36, 37]. Here, we discuss the use of radiation in young patients with TNBC. Few studies evaluating adjuvant radiotherapy have been conducted exclusively in young women with breast cancer, and most lack specifics about patients with TNBC. Beadle et al. [38] conducted a retrospective study to evaluate the impact of BCS, mastectomy alone, or mastectomy plus adjuvant radiotherapy on local recurrence rates in 652 patients ≤35 years, approximately 40% of whom had TNBC. After a median follow-up period of 114 months, the 10-year actuarial local recurrence rates in the entire cohort were 20% for BCS, 24% for mastectomy, and 15% for mastectomy plus adjuvant radiotherapy. When divided by disease stage, patients with stage II disease achieved the best locoregional control rates with mastectomy plus adjuvant radiotherapy. These results were promising, but the study had several limitations as it was a retrospective review and did not include a cohort of patients who had received BCS plus adjuvant radiation. Combination treatment is especially important for young women, as their absolute risk of local recurrence is higher than for older women [39, 40].

Minimizing the toxicities of radiotherapy in all younger cancer patients is especially important. Given that younger women with TNBC often present with larger, high-grade, node-positive tumors, this can be especially challenging as larger fields and higher doses may be needed. The potential toxicities of adjuvant radiation are well described [41] and include cardiac toxicity, pneumonitis, rib fractures, poor cosmesis, brachial plexopathy, and lymphedema, which can have long-term adverse effects on general health and QOL, particularly for women who will live decades after treatment. Cardiac toxicity is a major concern because most young patients with TNBC also receive anthracycline-based chemotherapy. Standard whole breast irradiation usually entails 6–7 weeks of daily radiation treatments (average doses 45–50 Gy), followed by a 10–16 Gy boost to the lumpectomy cavity for many women to further decrease local recurrence rates [42].

Newer techniques such as accelerated partial breast irradiation (APBI), dose hypofractionation, and proton therapy may reduce the side effects of radiation going forward, but few studies of these techniques have included many young women to date, and it is unclear if young women with TNBC can be safely treated this way. In fact, all consensus statements regarding APBI selection criteria [43, 44] include a minimum patient age ranging from 45 to 60 years due to the increased risk of multifocal and multicentric disease in young women, which may not be adequately treated with APBI. Similarly, hypofractionation is only recommended for women ≥50 years due to inadequate proof of safety and efficacy in younger patients [45]. With regard to boost radiation dosing, which carries added toxicity, the greatest benefit has been seen in women under 40 [46]. Until further evidence is available, standard of care for younger patients with breast cancer, including those with TNBC, remains delivery of whole-breast radiation with standard fractionation and consideration of a radiation boost.

10.2.3 Underuse of Radiation Therapy in Young Women with Breast Cancer

As discussed above, adjuvant radiation reduces the risk of local recurrence and improves breast cancer-specific survival in young women, including those with TNBC. However, lower compliance rates have been described in this subgroup [47]. Freedman et al. reported that younger women were less likely to receive radiation if BCS was performed. Uptake of radiotherapy was 69%, 73%, and 80% for women ≤35 years, 36–40 years, and 61–64 years, respectively [48]. Another study focusing on radiation in breast cancer patients who had BCS noted that 81% of women aged 50–55 years received adjuvant radiotherapy vs. 75% of women ≤35 years ($P < 0.0001$) [49]. Pan et al. [47] noted that women aged 20–50 years were less likely to receive radiotherapy than older patients. Having at least one child aged <7 years resulted in lower odds of receiving radiotherapy when compared with patients with no children or older children (7–12 years OR, 1.32; 95% CI, 1.05–1.66, $P < 0.02$; no children or children ≥18 years OR, 1.38; 95% CI, 1.13–1.68, $P < 0.001$) [47]. Other factors associated with a reduced likelihood of post-lumpectomy radiation included insurance type and distance to the radiation center. Geographic variations in compliance were also observed. Given that adjuvant radiation is a key component of the treatment for many young women with TNBC, the benefits should be carefully discussed prior to treatment initiation, which may improve compliance. Further, a social work consult may be valuable to young mothers who need financial and/or practical assistance with childcare.

10.2.4 Chemotherapy

Young women with TNBC are more likely to present with advanced disease, and the majority require chemotherapy. Fortunately, young patients are usually fit, with few comorbidities, and are therefore likely to tolerate treatment and derive benefit. Anthracycline/alkylator and taxane-based regimens are standard of care. In high-risk patients, dose-dense regimens using both anthracycline/alkylator and taxanes are preferred in the curative intent setting [50]. Approximately 20–30% of patients achieve a pathologic complete response (pCR), defined as no residual invasive cancer in either the excised tumor or lymph nodes, following neoadjuvant treatment [51, 52], which is a favorable prognostic factor [53, 54]. Interestingly, age seems to impact the chance of achieving pCR in this subtype of breast cancer, with higher rates of pCR among women <40 years (39.3%), compared to those aged 40–49 (37%) or ≥50 (25.2%) (*P* < 0.001) [55].

Treatment options for young TNBC patients who do not achieve pCR after neo-adjuvant chemotherapy include adjuvant capecitabine per the phase III CREATE-X study or participation in a clinical trial. In CREATE-X, 910 Japanese and Korean patients with HER2-negative residual invasive cancer after anthracycline- and/or taxane-based neoadjuvant chemotherapy were randomized to radiotherapy +/− endocrine therapy with or without 8 cycles of capecitabine (1250 mg/m^2 bid, days 1–14, every 3 weeks) [56]. Median patient age was only 48. DFS at 2 years was 87.3% for the capecitabine arm and 80.5% for patients who did not receive capecitabine (*P* = 0.001). There was also a trend toward improved OS at 2 years in the capecitabine-treated group at 96.2% and non-treated group at 93.9% (*P* = 0.086). In the capecitabine arm, grade 3 and 4 toxicities included hand-foot syndrome (11%), neutropenia (9%), diarrhea (3%), and fatigue (1%).Younger patients with TNBC may tolerate this regimen better than older patients, though this requires further study, and efficacy data are needed in non-Asian populations.

10.2.5 Fertility

Fertility preservation is an important issue for many young women with TNBC, as many require gonadotoxic chemotherapy. As women postpone childbearing for professional, cultural, and societal reasons [57], an increasing number of women diagnosed with TNBC have not completed their families and have concerns about treatment-related infertility [58]. With advances in reproductive endocrinology [59], options for fertility preservation are increasingly available [58], including ovarian function suppression (OFS), oocyte cryopreservation, and embryo cryopreservation [60]. The latter two are gold standard approaches, while the efficacy of OFS remains controversial. Ovarian tissue cryopreservation is also offered in an experimental fashion to women at select institutions. However, a significant number of women are not referred for fertility evaluation in a timely fashion [61], and others are not referred at all [62, 63]. Most comprehensive cancer centers do not have a formal protocol for the routine referral of young cancer patients to reproductive endocrinology [64].

The risk of infertility varies due to age, reproductive reserve, the chemotherapy agent used, and duration of treatment [65–67]. Alkylating agents are among those with the highest gonadotoxic properties [68–70]. Most young women with TNBC will require treatment with an alkylating agent, such as cyclophosphamide. Roughly 10–20% of women ≤35 who receive adjuvant chemotherapy for breast cancer develop permanent amenorrhea, but this risk rises with age to approximately 50% for a woman who is 40 years old at the time of chemotherapy initiation [66]. Further, *BRCA1* carriers may be more likely to have reduced ovarian reserve at the time of diagnosis, increasing the risk of premature menopause [71]. As 40% of women who develop TNBC ≤40 years carry a deleterious mutation in *BRCA1*, this is an important consideration when counseling these patients. True rates of infertility after breast cancer treatments have been difficult to ascertain [72], partly due to the heterogeneity of outcomes used to assess posttreatment ovarian function which include amenorrhea, follicle-stimulating hormone, serum estradiol, anti-Mullerian hormone, inhibin B, and antral follicle count [40].

There are many barriers to fertility preservation in young breast cancer patients despite the fact that concern about infertility causes substantial short- and long-term distress for young women diagnosed with breast cancer [73, 74]. Given that TNBC can behave aggressively and younger patients often present with locally advanced disease, it is possible that patients and/or their providers are wary about delaying systemic therapy to allow for fertility preservation in this setting. In a study assessing fertility concerns in 620 women with newly diagnosed early-stage breast cancer aged ≤40 years, non-white, childless patients and those advised to have chemotherapy expressed the greatest fertility concerns. A small number of women even declined or opted for suboptimal therapy given the infertility risk associated with gonadotoxic cancer treatments. These findings are especially relevant because TNBC is commonly seen in younger, African American women, in whom the majority will require chemotherapy. Furthermore, even though 51% reported fertility concerns, only 10% ultimately pursued assisted reproductive techniques [75]. Fertile Hope Centers of Excellence offers assistance to cancer patients who need financial and practical support [76, 77].

Data regarding the efficacy of gonadotropin-releasing hormone (GnRH) agonists in preserving ovarian function are mixed, and there is limited information regarding pregnancy outcomes [78]. In the Prevention of Early Menopause Study (POEMS) trial, 257 premenopausal women with operable hormone receptor-negative breast cancer were randomized to standard chemotherapy with the GnRH agonist goserelin or standard chemotherapy alone [79]. The primary endpoint was the rate of ovarian failure at 2 years. Secondary endpoints included pregnancy outcomes, DFS, and OS. Among 135 evaluable patients, the ovarian failure rate was 8% in the goserelin group and 22% in the chemotherapy-alone group ($P < 0.04$). Of 218 evaluable patients, more women became pregnant in the goserelin group than in the chemotherapy-alone group (21% vs. 11%, $P < 0.03$); women in the goserelin group also had improved DFS ($P < 0.04$) and OS ($P < 0.05$). Despite the large amount of missing data, this study suggests that there may be a reduction in risk of ovarian failure and premature menopause associated with the administration of goserelin before and during chemotherapy for young women with TNBC. This relatively simple intervention may be a good choice for young women with TNBC who cannot pursue assisted reproductive techniques due to financial, practical, or religious reasons.

10.2.6 Menopausal Symptoms

In addition to the implications for fertility, consequences of premature menopause include increased risks for osteoporosis, cardiovascular disease, cognitive decline, and dementia [80]. Given that premature menopause is a risk factor for osteoporosis, fragility fractures, and osteopenia, young patients with TNBC and additional risk factors could consider adjuvant bisphosphonate therapy [40]. However, women who have not completed childbearing are unsuitable candidates for bisphosphonates due to the potential embryotoxicity of these agents [81].

10.2.7 Contraception

Most young women need contraceptive counseling after a breast cancer diagnosis [82]. Hormonal methods of contraception are not recommended in breast cancer patients, including women with TNBC. Contraceptive methods utilized by young breast cancer patients are often insufficient, resulting in an increased risk of an unwanted pregnancy. In a cohort of young breast cancer patients during the first year after diagnosis ($\leq$40 years; $n = 100$), 62% of patients were either not using contraception or were using an ineffective method [83]. In the same study, 101 medical oncologists were surveyed with the aim of evaluating attitudes toward contraception in young breast cancer survivors. Almost all oncologists (99%) who responded to the survey believed that contraception is an important aspect in the surveillance of young patients with breast cancer, and the majority (90%) discussed the topic before commencing therapy. However, only 20% of the respondents discussed contraceptive methods during ongoing treatment and referred their patients for specialist counseling by a gynecologist. These findings are very concerning as chemotherapy is contraindicated during the first trimester of pregnancy. Therefore, an unplanned pregnancy can be devastating for young women recently diagnosed with breast cancer. Given the complexity of this topic, referral of young breast cancer patients to a gynecologist for specialist counseling may be advisable.

10.2.8 Childbearing After a Breast Cancer Diagnosis

No study to our knowledge has assessed maternal and fetal outcomes after treatment for TNBC specifically. Most evidence consists of case reports and retrospective cohort studies after breast cancer more generally. These studies may have a degree of selection bias, i.e., the "healthy mother" effect, in which women who become pregnant after breast cancer are healthier and less likely to develop a recurrence, whether they attempt pregnancy or not [84]. A large meta-analysis reported a 41% decreased mortality risk among women who become pregnant after their diagnosis compared with women who did not, especially in women with node-negative disease [85]. Although there is no evidence that pregnancy after breast cancer increases the risk of recurrent disease in the mother or congenital abnormalities in the fetus [86, 87], some women may avoid pregnancy due to concerns regarding both issues. However, survivors of TNBC are likely less concerned about the theoretical detrimental impact of pregnancy-associated hormonal fluctuations on recurrence risk than survivors of estrogen receptor-positive cancers [88, 89].

Nevertheless, as approximately 40% of young women with TNBC carry a deleterious mutation in *BRCA1*, this may affect attitudes toward future childbearing. Advances in reproductive endocrinology, preimplantation genetic diagnosis (PGD), and prenatal diagnosis (PND) are now options. A cross-sectional survey of 1081 *BRCA1/2* carriers assessed how knowledge of *BRCA* status influenced reproductive decision-making [90]. Mean age at *BRCA* test disclosure was 44 years, and 36% of women had a personal history of cancer. Of 163 single women, 21.5% felt greater pressure to get married. Of 284 women who desired future childbearing, 41% responded that carrier status influenced their decision to have biological children. Women with a history of cancer were more likely to report that knowledge of their *BRCA*-positive status impacted their decision to attempt a future pregnancy. About 59% and 55.5%, respectively, thought PGD and PND should be offered to *gBRCAm* carriers. Therefore, knowledge of *gBRCAm* status influences attitudes regarding relationships and childbearing, and most carriers think that PGD and PND should be an option for other carriers. This study implies that *gBRCAm* carriers would benefit from reproductive counseling after test disclosure.

10.3   Psychosocial Issues

Young women with TNBC often face greater psychosocial challenges than postmenopausal women. Fertility, body image issues, and lack of social support are associated with high levels of distress [35]. Furthermore, some young women decline recommended therapies due to their belief systems, lack of insurance, poor social support, or difficulty coping with the diagnosis, which ultimately increases their risk of local or distant recurrence. When Turkman and colleagues interviewed 22 TNBC patients aged ≤60, the central theme was the perception of TNBC as "an addendum" and "different" to other subtypes of breast cancer [91]. Other common themes included difficulty with decision-making, insecurity, and intense uncertainty. The authors concluded that most of the psychosocial needs of women with TNBC were unmet and have distinctive characteristics when compared to other breast cancer subtypes. Given the unique features of TNBC and the vulnerable populations disproportionately affected, further research studies should be conducted.

10.3.1   Effects in Quality of Life and Behaviors

Younger women with breast cancer report worse mental health-related QOL than both age-matched women without breast cancer and older women with breast cancer [92]. These patients may experience elevated levels of distress and depression following their diagnosis, which may persist into the survivorship phase [93]. A retrospective study in 577 breast cancer survivors who were <50 years at diagnosis noted that women ≤35 years old reported more emotional distress and less energy than older survivors, even years after initial treatment [94]. As TNBC is overrepresented in younger patients and is associated with inferior outcomes, rates of anxiety and depression may be greater in this subpopulation of breast cancer patients. TNBC treatment can impact diet, exercise, body image, work, recreation, finances, relationships, and sexuality. Younger women are more susceptible because they undergo more aggressive treatment. Fear of recurrence can also affect young TNBC patients' QOL after the conclusion of treatment and limit their ability to resume work and social activities. Importantly, despite the negative associations, a breast cancer diagnosis at a young age can be transformative. A unique phenomenon described in young cancer patients is their ability to find the "silver lining," making positive changes and developing a deepened appreciation for life [95].

10.3.2 Social Consequences

A breast cancer diagnosis at a young age can be a traumatic and disruptive life event. A young woman who does not know another breast cancer patient of a similar age may feel isolated and overwhelmed. She may have trouble relating to her peers given unique concerns about body image, appearance, dating, fertility, premature menopause, finances, childcare, and the risk of recurrence. Moreover, friends and co-workers may not know how to provide effective support, such that even well-intentioned friends end up avoiding the young woman with breast cancer [96]. Given that approximately 40% of women aged ≤40 with TNBC have a deleterious *BRCA1*, these women are additionally faced with the prospect of further preventative surgeries and the worry that they may have passed the mutation on to their children. In a focus group study of 36 young women with breast cancer, the average age was 37.8 years, and median time since diagnosis was approximately 2 years. The major themes that emerged were that participants felt different than older women with breast cancer diagnoses, had difficulty navigating the transition to survivorship, and desired connections both with other survivors and additional professionals including counselors [97]. Good social support is known to be associated with better adjustment after a breast cancer diagnosis, as well as increasing the likelihood of remaining at work while receiving treatment [98]. In a qualitative interview study of 20 breast cancer patients aged ≤42 (25% Hispanic, 15% black, 50% non-Hispanic whites, and 10% another race/ethnicity), similar needs for support and education were identified across various ethnicities [99]. Therefore, oncologists should provide relevant educational materials and consider early referral to support services. The Young Survival Coalition [100] is an international organization focused on increasing awareness and providing resources for women diagnosed with breast cancer aged <40 years. They can assist young women to find local support groups and community events aimed at young breast cancer patients, which may reduce the sense of isolation experienced by these young women.

A breast cancer diagnosis at a young age can adversely affect a woman's sexual functioning. Young breast cancer survivors in relationships are less sexually active and have more body image and sexual problems than similarly aged healthy women or older women with breast cancer [101]. A large prospective study surveyed 461 young women 1 year post-diagnosis of breast cancer about sexual functioning and interest, menopausal symptoms, amenorrhea, and somatic symptoms. Sexual functioning and interest were evaluated using the Cancer Rehabilitation Evaluation System (CARES) Sexual Functioning Summary Scale. Results showed that women with treatment-related amenorrhea experienced significantly decreased sexual interest and increased sexual dysfunction when compared to women without amenorrhea ($P < 0.002$). In multivariate analysis, body image, weight issues, and vaginal pain were independently associated with decreased sexual interest [35, 81, 98]. Relationship, sexual, and body image problems are clearly associated with reduced QOL in young breast cancer survivors [93].

Compared to older women, young breast cancer patients are less likely to have a well-established relationship at the time of diagnosis. For young women in a relationship, both partners may experience intense fear and anxiety, as the assumption of a long life together is called into question [35]. Multiple trips to the hospital and long chemotherapy infusions can result in severely disrupted routines and high stress levels, ultimately damaging the relationship. A recent study surveyed 491 women aged <45 years with non-metastatic breast cancer and their partners to identify differences in perceptions of their QOL during treatment and the active surveillance period. Patients reported greater difficulties with coping, finances, childcare, body image, and sexuality than their partners [102]. Conversely, single women may experience anxiety about pursuing intimate relationships, as the diagnosis takes up precious time that might otherwise have been used to establish an adult relationship and start a family [35]. In one study, young women who were married or had a stable partner were less likely to experience emotional distress after a cancer diagnosis [103].

Each young woman diagnosed with breast cancer will experience her own personal concerns. The experience of a college student diagnosed with breast cancer in her early 20s is different from that of a mother of teenage children in her early 40s. However, the emotional, educational, professional, and reproductive issues may be similar and be independent of chronological age [35, 104]. The ability to accept the cancer diagnosis, complete treatment, and continue with education or work may be related to emotional maturity and financial resources. Even in females with the same chronologic age, differences may be seen, from the 20-year-old female with a family history of breast cancer and a *gBRCA1m* to the childhood lymphoma survivor who underwent thoracic radiation and who may be more familiar with the medical system [104].

As previously mentioned, TNBC is overrepresented in young African American females. An integrative review identified that key psychosocial concerns for these women include anxiety, depression, relationships, and changes in cognition [105]. In a retrospective study of 355 African American females with breast cancer (median age 43.0), women with TNBC had an inferior QOL compared with those with other breast cancer subtypes ($P < 0.05$) [106]. Additionally, a systematic review of health-related quality of life (HRQOL) in younger black breast cancer survivors demonstrated that, when compared with their older, white, and breast cancer-free counterparts, these women reported lower physical and functional well-being, unmet supportive care needs, financial concerns, and greater fear of dying. Future research should focus on improving QOL measures in this vulnerable patient population [107].

10.3.3 Healthcare Disparities and Outcomes Across Ethnic Groups in Women with Triple-Negative Breast Cancer

It is well described that younger women with TNBC have inferior outcomes when compared with their older counterparts [108]. Young African American and Hispanic women with TNBC have even less favorable outcomes. In a retrospective study of 102,064 women aged ≥20, African American and American Indian/Alaska Native women had the greatest risk of being diagnosed with stage IV TNBC [109]. African American and Hispanic women were also at greater risk of not receiving guideline-concordant treatment. Globally, TNBC is more commonly seen in African American women as well as western, sub-Saharan African women. In a study of 223 Ghanaian breast cancer patients (median age 52.4 years), most women had palpable tumors >5 cm, and >50% had TNBC [110]. Patients also tended to have advanced stage disease and a younger age at diagnosis compared to Caucasian-Americans and African Americans. Also, many of these women may not have access to appropriate care given cultural, societal, financial and geographic issues. Overcoming boundaries to healthcare, as well as evaluating differences in reproductive, lifestyle, and dietary factors from genetic contributions to breast cancer disparities, is difficult [111]. Studying breast cancer risk related to ethnic identity is complex given epigenetics and experiences of societal inequality. Hopefully, further research into the molecular pathogenesis of TNBC will identify why it is more prevalent in women of African descent.

Conclusion

Relevant issues in the management of young women with TNBC include adverse tumor biology, diagnostic challenges, and increased likelihood of being a carrier of a genetic mutation, in addition to concerns regarding premature menopause, sexual functioning, infertility, and other long-term treatment-related toxicities. Future research should focus on healthcare disparities and psychosocial concerns relevant to younger women with TNBC, as many may benefit from additional psychological, social, and financial support at the time of diagnosis, during treatment, and into the survivorship period. We must ensure that young women are given accurate information regarding genetic testing, contraception, options for fertility preservation, and risks of treatment-related toxicities to optimize oncology outcomes and short- and long-term QOL in this vulnerable patient population.

References

1. Anders CK, Fan C, Parker JS, Carey LA, Blackwell KL, Klauber-DeMore N, et al. Breast carcinomas arising at a young age: unique biology or a surrogate for aggressive intrinsic subtypes? J Clin Oncol. 2011;29(1):e18–20.
2. American Cancer Society U. Breast Cancer Facts & Figures 2015–2016. 2016. https://www.cancer.org/content/dam/cancer-org/research/cancer-facts-and-statistics/breast-cancer-facts-and-figures/breast-cancer-facts-and-figures-2015-2016.pdf.

3. Liu Y, Xin T, Huang DY, Shen WX, Li L, Lv YJ, et al. Prognosis in very young women with triple-negative breast cancer: retrospective study of 216 cases. Med Oncol (Northwood, London, England). 2014;31(12):222.
4. Bleyer A, Barr R, Hayes-Lattin B, Thomas D, Ellis C, Anderson B, et al. The distinctive biology of cancer in adolescents and young adults. Nat Rev Cancer. 2008;8(4):288–98.
5. Anders CK, Johnson R, Litton J, Phillips M, Bleyer A. Breast cancer before age 40 years. Semin Oncol. 2009;36(3):237–49.
6. Han W, Kang SY. Relationship between age at diagnosis and outcome of premenopausal breast cancer: age less than 35 years is a reasonable cut-off for defining young age-onset breast cancer. Breast Cancer Res Treat. 2010;119(1):193–200.
7. Foxcroft LM, Evans EB, Porter AJ. The diagnosis of breast cancer in women younger than 40. Breast (Edinburgh, Scotland). 2004;13(4):297–306.
8. Yao Y, Cao M, Fang H, Xie J. Breast cancer in 30-year-old or younger patients: clinicopathologic characteristics and prognosis. World J Surg Oncol. 2015;13:38.
9. Barber MD, Jack W, Dixon JM. Diagnostic delay in breast cancer. Br J Surg. 2004;91(1):49–53.
10. Jassem J, Ozmen V, Bacanu F, Drobniene M, Eglitis J, Lakshmaiah KC, et al. Delays in diagnosis and treatment of breast cancer: a multinational analysis. Eur J Pub Health. 2014;24(5):761–7.
11. Axelrod D, Smith J, Kornreich D, Grinstead E, Singh B, Cangiarella J, et al. Breast cancer in young women. J Am Coll Surg. 2008;206(6):1193–203.
12. Ruddy KJ, Gelber S, Tamimi RM, Schapira L, Come SE, Meyer ME, et al. Breast cancer presentation and diagnostic delays in young women. Cancer. 2014;120(1):20–5.
13. Colak D, Nofal A, Albakheet A, Nirmal M, Jeprel H, Eldali A, et al. Age-specific gene expression signatures for breast tumors and cross-species conserved potential cancer progression markers in young women. PLoS One. 2013;8(5):e63204.
14. Yau C, Fedele V, Roydasgupta R, Fridlyand J, Hubbard A, Gray JW, et al. Aging impacts transcriptomes but not genomes of hormone-dependent breast cancers. Breast Cancer Res. 2007;9(5):R59.
15. Dai H, van't Veer L, Lamb J, He YD, Mao M, Fine BM, et al. A cell proliferation signature is a marker of extremely poor outcome in a subpopulation of breast cancer patients. Cancer Res. 2005;65(10):4059–66.
16. Quong J, Eppenberger-Castori S, Moore D 3rd, Scott GK, Birrer MJ, Kueng W, et al. Age-dependent changes in breast cancer hormone receptors and oxidant stress markers. Breast Cancer Res Treat. 2002;76(3):221–36.
17. Anders CK, Hsu DS, Broadwater G, Acharya CR, Foekens JA, Zhang Y, et al. Young age at diagnosis correlates with worse prognosis and defines a subset of breast cancers with shared patterns of gene expression. J Clin Oncol. 2008;26(20):3324–30.
18. Daly MB, Pilarski R, Berry M, Buys SS, Farmer M, Friedman S, et al. NCCN guidelines insights: genetic/familial high-risk assessment: breast and ovarian, version 2.2017. J Natl Compr Cancer Netw. 2017;15(1):9–20.
19. Atchley DP, Albarracin CT, Lopez A, Valero V, Amos CI, Gonzalez-Angulo AM, et al. Clinical and pathologic characteristics of patients with BRCA-positive and BRCA-negative breast cancer. J Clin Oncol. 2008;26(26):4282–8.
20. Comen E, Davids M, Kirchhoff T, Hudis C, Offit K, Robson M. Relative contributions of BRCA1 and BRCA2 mutations to "triple-negative" breast cancer in Ashkenazi Women. Breast Cancer Res Treat. 2011;129(1):185–90.
21. van den Broek AJ, van't Veer LJ, Hooning MJ, Cornelissen S, Broeks A, Rutgers EJ, et al. Impact of age at primary breast cancer on contralateral breast cancer risk in BRCA1/2 mutation carriers. J Clin Oncol. 2016;34(5):409–18.
22. Malone KE, Begg CB, Haile RW, Borg A, Concannon P, Tellhed L, et al. Population-based study of the risk of second primary contralateral breast cancer associated with carrying a mutation in BRCA1 or BRCA2. J Clin Oncol. 2010;28(14):2404–10.
23. Graeser MK, Engel C, Rhiem K, Gadzicki D, Bick U, Kast K, et al. Contralateral breast cancer risk in BRCA1 and BRCA2 mutation carriers. J Clin Oncol. 2009;27(35):5887–92.

24. Metcalfe KA, Birenbaum-Carmeli D, Lubinski J, Gronwald J, Lynch H, Moller P, et al. International variation in rates of uptake of preventive options in BRCA1 and BRCA2 mutation carriers. Int J Cancer. 2008;122(9):2017–22.
25. Gonzalez-Angulo AM, Timms KM, Liu S, Chen H, Litton JK, Potter J, et al. Incidence and outcome of BRCA mutations in unselected patients with triple receptor-negative breast cancer. Clin Cancer Res. 2011;17(5):1082–9.
26. Habermann EB, Abbott A, Parsons HM, Virnig BA, Al-Refaie WB, Tuttle TM. Are mastectomy rates really increasing in the United States? J Clin Oncol. 2010;28(21):3437–41.
27. Middleton LP, Amin M, Gwyn K, Theriault R, Sahin A. Breast carcinoma in pregnant women: assessment of clinicopathologic and immunohistochemical features. Cancer. 2003;98(5):1055–60.
28. Couch FJ, Hart SN, Sharma P, Toland AE, Wang X, Miron P, et al. Inherited mutations in 17 breast cancer susceptibility genes among a large triple-negative breast cancer cohort unselected for family history of breast cancer. J Clin Oncol. 2015;33(4):304–11.
29. Domagala P, Jakubowska A, Jaworska-Bieniek K, Kaczmarek K, Durda K, Kurlapska A, et al. Prevalence of germline mutations in genes engaged in DNA damage repair by homologous recombination in patients with triple-negative and hereditary non-triple-negative breast cancers. PLoS One. 2015;10(6):e0130393.
30. Baptiste DF, MacGeorge EL, Venetis MK, Mouton A, Friley LB, Pastor R, et al. Motivations for contralateral prophylactic mastectomy as a function of socioeconomic status. BMC Womens Health. 2017;17(1):10.
31. Rakovitch E, Franssen E, Kim J, Ackerman I, Pignol JP, Paszat L, et al. A comparison of risk perception and psychological morbidity in women with ductal carcinoma in situ and early invasive breast cancer. Breast Cancer Res Treat. 2003;77(3):285–93.
32. Rosenberg SM, Tracy MS, Meyer ME, Sepucha K, Gelber S, Hirshfield-Bartek J, et al. Perceptions, knowledge, and satisfaction with contralateral prophylactic mastectomy among young women with breast cancer: a cross-sectional survey. Ann Intern Med. 2013;159(6):373–81.
33. Fisher CS, Martin-Dunlap T, Ruppel MB, Gao F, Atkins J, Margenthaler JA. Fear of recurrence and perceived survival benefit are primary motivators for choosing mastectomy over breast-conservation therapy regardless of age. Ann Surg Oncol. 2012;19(10):3246–50.
34. Abbott A, Rueth N, Pappas-Varco S, Kuntz K, Kerr E, Tuttle T. Perceptions of contralateral breast cancer: an overestimation of risk. Ann Surg Oncol. 2011;18(11):3129–36.
35. Ganz PA, Kwan L, Stanton AL, Krupnick JL, Rowland JH, Meyerowitz BE, et al. Quality of life at the end of primary treatment of breast cancer: first results from the moving beyond cancer randomized trial. J Natl Cancer Inst. 2004;96(5):376–87.
36. Freedman GM. Radiation therapy for operable breast cancer: sixty years of progress as seen through the articles published in the journal Cancer. Cancer. 2008;113(7 Suppl):1779–800.
37. Rustogi A, Budrukkar A, Dinshaw K, Jalali R. Management of locally advanced breast cancer: evolution and current practice. J Cancer Res Ther. 2005;1(1):21–30.
38. Beadle BM, Woodward WA, Tucker SL, Outlaw ED, Allen PK, JL O, et al. Ten-year recurrence rates in young women with breast cancer by locoregional treatment approach. Int J Radiat Oncol Biol Phys. 2009;73(3):734–44.
39. Early Breast Cancer Trialists' Collaborative G, Darby S, McGale P, Correa C, Taylor C, Arriagada R, et al. Effect of radiotherapy after breast-conserving surgery on 10-year recurrence and 15-year breast cancer death: meta-analysis of individual patient data for 10,801 women in 17 randomised trials. Lancet. 2011;378(9804):1707–16.
40. Ademuyiwa FO, Cyr A, Ivanovich J, Thomas MA. Managing breast cancer in younger women: challenges and solutions. Breast Cancer (Dove Med Press). 2016;8:1–12.
41. Speers C, Pierce LJ. Postoperative radiotherapy after breast-conserving surgery for early-stage breast cancer: a review. JAMA Oncol. 2016;2(8):1075–82.
42. Tann AW, Hatch SS, Joyner MM, Wiederhold LR, Swanson TA. Accelerated partial breast irradiation: past, present, and future. World J Clin Oncol. 2016;7(5):370–9.

43. Smith BD, Arthur DW, Buchholz TA, Haffty BG, Hahn CA, Hardenbergh PH, et al. Accelerated partial breast irradiation consensus statement from the American Society for Radiation Oncology (ASTRO). Int J Radiat Oncol Biol Phys. 2009;74(4):987–1001.
44. Shah C, Vicini F, Wazer DE, Arthur D, Patel RR. The American Brachytherapy Society consensus statement for accelerated partial breast irradiation. Brachytherapy. 2013;12(4):267–77.
45. Smith BD, Bentzen SM, Correa CR, Hahn CA, Hardenbergh PH, Ibbott GS, et al. Fractionation for whole breast irradiation: an American Society for Radiation Oncology (ASTRO) evidence-based guideline. Int J Radiat Oncol Biol Phys. 2011;81(1):59–68.
46. Bartelink H, Horiot JC, Poortmans P, Struikmans H, Van den Bogaert W, Barillot I, et al. Recurrence rates after treatment of breast cancer with standard radiotherapy with or without additional radiation. N Engl J Med. 2001;345(19):1378–87.
47. Pan IW, Smith BD, Shih YC. Factors contributing to underuse of radiation among younger women with breast cancer. J Natl Cancer Inst. 2014;106(1):djt340.
48. Freedman RA, Virgo KS, Labadie J, He Y, Partridge AH, Keating NL. Receipt of locoregional therapy among young women with breast cancer. Breast Cancer Res Treat. 2012;135(3):893–906.
49. Maggard MA, O'Connell JB, Lane KE, Liu JH, Etzioni DA, Ko CY. Do young breast cancer patients have worse outcomes? J Surg Res. 2003;113(1):109–13.
50. Citron ML, Berry DA, Cirrincione C, Hudis C, Winer EP, Gradishar WJ, et al. Randomized trial of dose-dense versus conventionally scheduled and sequential versus concurrent combination chemotherapy as postoperative adjuvant treatment of node-positive primary breast cancer: first report of Intergroup Trial C9741/Cancer and Leukemia Group B Trial 9741. J Clin Oncol. 2003;21(8):1431–9.
51. Liedtke C, Mazouni C, Hess KR, Andre F, Tordai A, Mejia JA, et al. Response to neoadjuvant therapy and long-term survival in patients with triple-negative breast cancer. J Clin Oncol. 2008;26(8):1275–81.
52. Sikov WM, Berry DA, Perou CM, Singh B, Cirrincione CT, Tolaney SM, et al. Impact of the addition of carboplatin and/or bevacizumab to neoadjuvant once-per-week paclitaxel followed by dose-dense doxorubicin and cyclophosphamide on pathologic complete response rates in stage II to III triple-negative breast cancer: CALGB 40603 (Alliance). J Clin Oncol. 2015;33(1):13–21.
53. von Minckwitz G, Untch M, Blohmer JU, Costa SD, Eidtmann H, Fasching PA, et al. Definition and impact of pathologic complete response on prognosis after neoadjuvant chemotherapy in various intrinsic breast cancer subtypes. J Clin Oncol. 2012;30(15):1796–804.
54. Cortazar P, Zhang L, Untch M, Mehta K, Costantino JP, Wolmark N, et al. Pathological complete response and long-term clinical benefit in breast cancer: the CTNeoBC pooled analysis. Lancet. 2014;384(9938):164–72.
55. Loibl S, Jackisch C, Lederer B, Untch M, Paepke S, Kummel S, et al. Outcome after neoadjuvant chemotherapy in young breast cancer patients: a pooled analysis of individual patient data from eight prospectively randomized controlled trials. Breast Cancer Res Treat. 2015;152(2):377–87.
56. Masuda N, Lee S-J, Ohtani S, Im Y-H, Lee E-S, Yokota I, et al. Adjuvant capecitabine for breast cancer after preoperative chemotherapy. N Engl J Med. 2017;376(22):2147–59.
57. Cooke A, Mills TA, Lavender T. 'Informed and uninformed decision making'—women's reasoning, experiences and perceptions with regard to advanced maternal age and delayed childbearing: a meta-synthesis. Int J Nurs Stud. 2010;47:1317–29.
58. Loren AW, Mangu PB, Beck LN, Brennan L, Magdalinski AJ, Partridge AH, et al. Fertility preservation for patients with cancer: american society of clinical oncology clinical practice guideline update. J Clin Oncol. 2013;31:2500–10.
59. Moragianni VA, Penzias AS. Cumulative live-birth rates after assisted reproductive technology. Curr Opin Obstet Gynecol. 2010;22(3):189–92.
60. Waks AG, Partridge AH. Fertility preservation in patients with breast cancer: necessity, methods, and safety. J Natl Compr Cancer Netw. 2016;14(3):355–63.

61. Lee S, Ozkavukcu S, Heytens E, Moy F, Oktay K. Value of early referral to fertility preservation in young women with breast cancer. J Clin Oncol. 2010;28(31):4683–6.
62. Quinn GP, Vadaparampil ST, Lee JH, Jacobsen PB, Bepler G, Lancaster J, et al. Physician referral for fertility preservation in oncology patients: a national study of practice behaviors. J Clin Oncol. 2009;27:5952–7.
63. Banerjee R, Tsiapali E. Occurrence and recall rates of fertility discussions with young breast cancer patients. Support Care Cancer. 2016;24(1):163–71.
64. Clayman ML, Harper MM, Quinn GP, Reinecke J, Shah S. Oncofertility resources at NCI-designated comprehensive cancer centers. J Natl Compr Cancer Netw. 2013;11(12):1504–9.
65. Azim HA Jr, de Azambuja E, Colozza M, Bines J, Piccart MJ. Long-term toxic effects of adjuvant chemotherapy in breast cancer. Ann Oncol. 2011;22(9):1939–47.
66. Abusief ME, Missmer SA, Ginsburg ES, Weeks JC, Partridge AH. The effects of paclitaxel, dose density, and trastuzumab on treatment-related amenorrhea in premenopausal women with breast cancer. Cancer. 2010;116(4):791–8.
67. Walshe JM, Denduluri N, Swain SM. Amenorrhea in premenopausal women after adjuvant chemotherapy for breast cancer. J Clin Oncol. 2006;24(36):5769–79.
68. Levine JM, Kelvin JF, Quinn GP, Gracia CR. Infertility in reproductive-age female cancer survivors. Cancer. 2015;121(10):1532–9.
69. Zhou WB, Yin H, Liu XA, Zha XM, Chen L, Dai JC, et al. Incidence of chemotherapy-induced amenorrhea associated with epirubicin, docetaxel and navelbine in younger breast cancer patients. BMC Cancer. 2010;10:281.
70. Parulekar WR, Day AG, Ottaway JA, Shepherd LE, Trudeau ME, Bramwell V, et al. Incidence and prognostic impact of amenorrhea during adjuvant therapy in high-risk premenopausal breast cancer: analysis of a National Cancer Institute of Canada Clinical Trials Group Study—NCIC CTG MA.5. J Clin Oncol. 2005;23(25):6002–8.
71. Titus S, Li F, Stobezki R, Akula K, Unsal E, Jeong K, et al. Impairment of BRCA1-related DNA double-strand break repair leads to ovarian aging in mice and humans. Sci Transl Med. 2013;5(172):172ra21.
72. Oktay K, Oktem O, Reh A, Vahdat L. Measuring the impact of chemotherapy on fertility in women with breast cancer. J Clin Oncol. 2006;24(24):4044–6.
73. Partridge AH, Ruddy KJ, Kennedy J, Winer EP. Model program to improve care for a unique cancer population: young women with breast cancer. J Oncol Pract. 2012;8(5):e105–10.
74. Senkus E, Gomez H, Dirix L, Jerusalem G, Murray E, Van Tienhoven G, et al. Attitudes of young patients with breast cancer toward fertility loss related to adjuvant systemic therapies. EORTC study 10002 BIG 3-98. Psycho-Oncology. 2014;23(2):173–82.
75. Ruddy KJ, Gelber SI, Tamimi RM, Ginsburg ES, Schapira L, Come SE, et al. Prospective study of fertility concerns and preservation strategies in young women with breast cancer. J Clin Oncol. 2014;32(11):1151–6.
76. Reinecke JD, Kelvin JF, Arvey SR, Quinn GP, Levine J, Beck LN, et al. Implementing a systematic approach to meeting patients' cancer and fertility needs: a review of the Fertile Hope Centers of Excellence program. J Oncol Pract. 2012;8(5):303–8.
77. Shay LA, Parsons HM, Vernon SW. Survivorship care planning and unmet information and service needs among adolescent and young adult cancer survivors. J Adolesc Young Adult Oncol. 2017.
78. Del Mastro L, Catzeddu T, Venturini M. Infertility and pregnancy after breast cancer: current knowledge and future perspectives. Cancer Treat Rev. 2006;32(6):417–22.
79. Moore HC, Unger JM, Phillips KA, Boyle F, Hitre E, Porter D, et al. Goserelin for ovarian protection during breast-cancer adjuvant chemotherapy. N Engl J Med. 2015;372(10):923–32.
80. Shuster LT, Rhodes DJ, Gostout BS, Grossardt BR, Rocca WA. Premature menopause or early menopause: long-term health consequences. Maturitas. 2010;65(2):161–6.
81. Ferzoco RM, Ruddy KJ. Unique aspects of caring for young breast cancer patients. Curr Oncol Rep. 2015;17(2):1.
82. Guth U, Huang DJ, Bitzer J, Tirri BF, Moffat R. Contraception counseling for young breast cancer patients: a practical needs assessment and a survey among medical oncologists. Breast (Edinburgh, Scotland). 2016;30:217–21.

83. Guth U, Huang DJ, Bitzer J, Moffat R. Unintended pregnancy during the first year after breast cancer diagnosis. Eur J Contracept Reprod Health Care. 2016;21(4):290–4.
84. Hartman EK, Eslick GD. The prognosis of women diagnosed with breast cancer before, during and after pregnancy: a meta-analysis. Breast Cancer Res Treat. 2016;160(2):347–60.
85. Raphael J, Trudeau ME, Chan K. Outcome of patients with pregnancy during or after breast cancer: a review of the recent literature. Curr Oncol. 2015;22(Suppl 1):S8–S18.
86. Mueller BA, Chow EJ, Kamineni A, Daling JR, Fraser A, Wiggins CL, et al. Pregnancy outcomes in female childhood and adolescent cancer survivors: a linked cancer-birth registry analysis. Arch Pediatr Adolesc Med. 2009;163(10):879–86.
87. Sankila R, Heinavaara S, Hakulinen T. Survival of breast cancer patients after subsequent term pregnancy: "healthy mother effect". Am J Obstet Gynecol. 1994;170(3):818–23.
88. Azim HA Jr, Santoro L, Pavlidis N, Gelber S, Kroman N, Azim H, et al. Safety of pregnancy following breast cancer diagnosis: a meta-analysis of 14 studies. Eur J Cancer. 2011;47:74–83.
89. Quinn GP, Vadaparampil ST, Bower B, Friedman S, Keefe DL. Decisions and ethical issues among BRCA carriers and the use of preimplantation genetic diagnosis. Minerva Med. 2009;100(5):371–83.
90. Chan JL, Johnson LN, Sammel MD, DiGiovanni L, Voong C, Domchek SM, et al. Reproductive decision-making in women with BRCA1/2 mutations. J Genet Couns. 2017;26(3):594–603.
91. Turkman YE, Kennedy HP, Harris LN, Knobf MT. "An addendum to breast cancer": the triple negative experience. Support Care Cancer. 2016;24(9):3715–21.
92. Champion VL, Wagner LI, Monahan PO, Daggy J, Smith L, Cohee A, et al. Comparison of younger and older breast cancer survivors and age-matched controls on specific and overall quality of life domains. Cancer. 2014;120(15):2237–46.
93. Avis NE, Levine B, Naughton MJ, Case DL, Naftalis E, Van Zee KJ. Explaining age-related differences in depression following breast cancer diagnosis and treatment. Breast Cancer Res Treat. 2012;136(2):581–91.
94. Wenzel LB, Fairclough DL, Brady MJ, Cella D, Garrett KM, Kluhsman BC, et al. Age-related differences in the quality of life of breast carcinoma patients after treatment. Cancer. 1999;86(9):1768–74.
95. Koutrouli N, Anagnostopoulos F, Potamianos G. Posttraumatic stress disorder and posttraumatic growth in breast cancer patients: a systematic review. Women Health. 2012;52(5):503–16.
96. Adams E, McCann L, Armes J, Richardson A, Stark D, Watson E, et al. The experiences, needs and concerns of younger women with breast cancer: a meta-ethnography. Psycho-Oncology. 2011;20(8):851–61.
97. Ruddy KJ, Greaney ML, Sprunck-Harrild K, Meyer ME, Emmons KM, Partridge AH. Young women with breast cancer: a focus group study of unmet needs. J Adolesc Young Adult Oncol. 2013;2(4):153–60.
98. Howard-Anderson J, Ganz PA, Bower JE, Stanton AL. Quality of life, fertility concerns, and behavioral health outcomes in younger breast cancer survivors: a systematic review. J Natl Cancer Inst. 2012;104(5):386–405.
99. Ruddy KJ, Greaney ML, Sprunck-Harrild K, Meyer ME, Emmons KM, Partridge AH. A qualitative exploration of supports and unmet needs of diverse young women with breast cancer. J Community Support Oncol. 2015;13(9):323–9.
100. Vento R, D'Alessandro N, Giuliano M, Lauricella M, Carabillo M, Tesoriere G. Induction of apoptosis by arachidonic acid in human retinoblastoma Y79 cells: involvement of oxidative stress. Exp Eye Res. 2000;70(4):503–17.
101. Fobair P, Stewart SL, Chang S, D'Onofrio C, Banks PJ, Bloom JR. Body image and sexual problems in young women with breast cancer. Psycho-Oncology. 2006;15(7):579–94.
102. Vanlemmens L, Fournier E, Boinon D, Machavoine JL, Christophe V. [Quality of life of young women with early breast cancer and their partners: specific needs result in the necessity of development of specific questionnaires for the patient and the partner]. Bull Cancer. 2012;99(6):685–691.

103. Baucom DH, Porter LS, Kirby JS, Gremore TM, Keefe FJ. Psychosocial issues confronting young women with breast cancer. Breast Dis. 2005;23:103–13.
104. Moskowitz CS, Chou JF, Wolden SL, Bernstein JL, Malhotra J, Novetsky Friedman D, et al. Breast cancer after chest radiation therapy for childhood cancer. J Clin Oncol. 2014;32(21):2217–23.
105. Nolan TS, Frank J, Gisiger-Camata S, Meneses K. An integrative review of psychosocial concerns among young African American breast cancer survivors. Cancer Nurs. 2017.
106. Vadaparampil ST, Christie J, Donovan KA, Kim J, Augusto B, Kasting ML, et al. Health-related quality of life in black breast cancer survivors with and without triple-negative breast cancer (TNBC). Breast Cancer Res Treat. 2017;163(2):331–42.
107. Samuel CA, Pinheiro LC, Reeder-Hayes KE, Walker JS, Corbie-Smith G, Fashaw SA, et al. To be young, black, and living with breast cancer: a systematic review of health-related quality of life in young black breast cancer survivors. Breast Cancer Res Treat. 2016;160(1):1–15.
108. Joyce DP, Murphy D, Lowery AJ, Curran C, Barry K, Malone C, et al. Prospective comparison of outcome after treatment for triple-negative and non-triple-negative breast cancer. Surgeon. 2017;15(5):272–7.
109. Chen L, Li CI. Racial disparities in breast cancer diagnosis and treatment by hormone receptor and HER2 status. Cancer Epidemiol Biomark Prev. 2015;24(11):1666–72.
110. Der EM, Gyasi RK, Tettey Y, Edusei L, Bayor MT, Jiagge E, et al. Triple-negative breast cancer in Ghanaian women: the Korle Bu Teaching Hospital experience. Breast J. 2015;21(6):627–33.
111. Newman LA, Kaljee LM. Health disparities and triple-negative breast cancer in African American women: a review. JAMA Surg. 2017;152(5):485–93.

Individualizing the Approach to the Older Woman with Triple-Negative Breast Cancer

Jasmeet Chadha Singh and Stuart M. Lichtman

Clinical Pearls
- For elderly patients with early-stage triple-negative breast cancer and a life expectancy more than 5 years, chemotherapy is the main systemic approach as older patients derive the same benefits from systemic therapies as their younger counterparts.
- Patients 70 years of age and older with early-stage triple-negative breast cancer should be offered the same breast surgery options as their younger counterparts.
- Appropriate geriatric assessment tools should be utilized when prescribing systemic therapies to elderly patients with triple-negative breast cancer.

11.1 Introduction

Advanced age is an important risk factor for breast cancer with about 21% of cases occurring in patients over 70 years of age [1]. The National Comprehensive Cancer Network (NCCN) has defined the elderly population as patients aged >65 years [2]. The triple-negative subtype is defined as breast cancer with absence of estrogen receptor (ER) and progesterone receptor (PR) staining by immunohistochemistry (IHC) and lack of human epidermal growth factor receptor type 2 (HER2)

J.C. Singh, MD (✉)
Breast Medicine Division, Department of Medicine, Memorial Sloan Kettering Cancer Center, West Harrison, NY, USA
e-mail: singhj@mskcc.org

S.M. Lichtman, MD
Weill Cornell Medical College, Memorial Sloan Kettering Cancer Center, Commack, NY, USA
e-mail: lichtmas@mskcc.org

© Springer International Publishing AG 2018
A.R. Tan (ed.), *Triple-Negative Breast Cancer*,
https://doi.org/10.1007/978-3-319-69980-6_11

expression by IHC and/or a fluorescent in situ hybridization (FISH) ratio of less than 2 [3]. It is an aggressive subtype of breast cancer and is usually more common in younger patients [4, 5]. Although elderly patients tend to have hormone receptor (HR)-positive tumors [6], about 18% of elderly women have triple-negative breast cancer (TNBC). Despite advances in anticancer therapies, elderly patients often receive insufficient local and systemic therapies [7–9].

11.2   Epidemiology and Clinical Presentation

TNBC accounts for about 15–20% of breast cancers diagnosed worldwide. Although it is more commonly seen in younger patients, about 19% of patients diagnosed with TNBC are older than 70 years of age [6]. TNBC is deemed to be an aggressive subtype of breast cancer, with higher incidence of local and distant recurrences and worse overall survival [10–12]. However, older-aged women tend to develop tumors that harbor a benign biological phenotype with a lower probability of lymph node metastasis, earlier TNM stage, and better differentiation. In a large case series at a single center, increasing age was associated with better disease-free survival (DFS) and overall survival (OS) in TNBC regardless of size, stage, and grade of tumor [13, 14].

11.3   Treatment Approach

While 49% of breast cancer occurs in elderly women, this population remains largely underrepresented in cooperative group therapeutic clinical trials [15, 16]. Only 3% of patients older than 70 years participate in clinical trials [17]. Hence, there is paucity of data regarding how to appropriately manage elderly patients with breast cancer.

Surgery is the main local therapy for early breast cancer; however, there is a concern regarding anesthesia and wound healing complications in elderly patients. Several studies have shown that elderly patients are often undertreated compared to their younger counterparts. In a study comparing local and systemic treatments for breast cancer in the following age groups of 70–74, 75–80, and >80, the latter subgroup received less extensive surgery, less adjuvant radiation therapy, and less chemotherapy [9]. In a Surveillance, Epidemiology, and End Results (SEER)-based population study involving 9908 women, elderly TNBC cases were associated with distinctly worse overall and cancer-specific survival than their young counterparts. The 18-month OS rate was 84.6% in the elderly group compared with 93.4% in the younger group. The 18-month cancer-specific survival rates were 91.0% and 94.3% in the elderly and younger groups, respectively, which suggested a survival disadvantage related to older age. It was also observed that a significant proportion of TNBC patients did not undergo surgery and/or radiation as a part of local treatment where it was indicated [14]. As per the International Society of Geriatric Oncology's (SIOG) recommendations, patients 70 years of age or older with early-stage breast cancer should be offered the same surgery as younger patients, namely, breast conservation surgery (BCS) with whole breast radiation therapy or mastectomy with or without breast reconstructive surgery. Elderly patients are less likely to choose immediate breast reconstruction; however, a review of the National Cancer Database records from 2004 to 2012 showed that the rate of mastectomy and ipsilateral breast reconstruction seems to be on the rise in patients who are 65 years of age and older [18].

Although there is data showing that radiation can be avoided in low-risk elderly patients with early-stage ER-positive breast cancer who undergo BCS, TNBC patients benefit from adjuvant radiation therapy [19, 20]. According to the SEER database analysis of elderly patients with T1–T2, N0M0 TNBC, lumpectomy and adjuvant radiation was associated with improved OS (98.2% versus 85.6%, P = <0.001) and disease-specific survival (99% versus 94%, P = 0.003) compared to lumpectomy alone [21].

Although the NCCN definition of elderly patients is age >65 years, it is usually the patients over 70 years who are at risk of complications of chemotherapy due to age-related comorbidities. In contrast to chronological aging, biological aging is heterogeneous. Patients who are in an excellent state of health at 75 years of age may have a life expectancy upward of 10 additional years [22]. Several factors make management of elderly patients more complicated than the younger ones [23]. These are described in the following section.

11.3.1 Comorbidities and Age-Related Changes Influencing Pharmacokinetics and Pharmacodynamics

Most pharmacokinetic studies have involved young, healthy patients without significant comorbidities. The pharmacokinetic differences with aging may not be great, but additive effects of multiple morbidities and end-organ dysfunction make these differences significant. Many older patients suffer from health-related conditions prior to their cancer diagnosis, which can make treatment with chemotherapy challenging. Patients with prior cardiopulmonary issues such as myocardial ischemia and heart failure may have increased toxicity from anthracycline-based regimens [24, 25]. Moreover, there is a well-documented decline in hepatic and renal function with aging which can predispose patients to toxicity [26–28]. Serum creatinine measurement by itself is not a reliable indicator of renal function in the older population, as renal dysfunction may exist despite normal serum creatinine. Age-related changes in splanchnic blood flow, motility, and mucosal atrophy result in changes in drug absorption [29–32].

11.3.2 Polypharmacy

Elderly patients are often on multiple medications which may interact with their chemotherapeutic drugs [33–35]. Moreover, the use of complimentary medications such as high-dose vitamins and herbal supplements is increasing among elderly patients. Studies have shown that the use of these supplements may enhance toxic effects of chemotherapy and reduce benefit via CYP metabolism and P-glycoprotein transport [36–40].

11.3.3 Cognitive Decline and Imbalance

Age-related cognitive decline may interfere with compliance [41, 42] and reporting of side effects and may increase frequency of falls leading to subsequent hospitalization.

11.4   Geriatric Assessment Tools

Online tools like Adjuvant Online are available to calculate adjuvant chemotherapy benefit. However, caution should be exercised while employing them for older patients as they do not take into account geriatric parameters such as comorbidities and performance status, thus leading to overtreatment and chemotherapy-related toxicities [43, 44].

Currently, SIOG and NCCN recommend performing geriatric assessment for elderly patients with cancer [45, 46]. There are clinical scores systematically integrating both chemotherapy and patient risk for older patients. The Chemotherapy Risk Assessment Scale for High-Age Patients (CRASH) score was constructed along two subscores determining hematologic (H) toxicity and non-hematologic (NH) toxicity. Variables predicting H toxicity were lymphocytes, aspartate aminotransferase level, Instrumental Activities of Daily Living score, lactate dehydrogenase level, diastolic blood pressure, and toxicity of chemotherapy regimen. Predictors of NH toxicity were hemoglobin, creatinine clearance, albumin, self-rated health, Eastern Cooperative Oncology Group performance, Mini-Mental State Examination score, Mini-Nutritional Assessment score, and chemotoxicity [47].

The Cancer and Aging Research Group (CARG) is another comprehensive tool which takes into account patients' age, tumor, treatment, lab values, and geriatric variables that helps identify deficits such as limitation in instrumental activities of daily living (IADLs), comorbidities, and polypharmacy in elderly who are deemed to have good performance status. This model was validated in a recent study of 250 patients, where a statistically significant difference in toxicity rates was observed in patients with low-medium and high score groups [48–50]. Early identification and intervention to correct these deficits helps in ameliorating these risk factors that could potentially complicate chemotherapy course by early intervention [51].

11.5   Adjuvant Chemotherapy

There is mounting evidence that elderly patients with high-risk disease who are not offered adjuvant chemotherapy have worse disease-specific survival [52]. However, there is a paucity of specific clinical trials establishing benefit of adjuvant chemotherapy in an older patient. The phase III ACTION trial designed to look at benefits of adjuvant chemotherapy with doxorubicin and cyclophosphamide (AC) versus observation in elderly patients with ER-negative or weakly positive breast cancer did not meet accrual goals [53]. There are studies suggesting that elderly patients with high-risk disease, when treated with adjuvant anthracycline chemotherapy, derive equal benefits compared to their younger counterparts. There is also an indication that elderly patients treated with aggressive chemotherapy have a better DFS compared to their younger counterparts. However, this comes at a cost of increased grade 3 or higher hematological toxicity [54].

The Early Breast Cancer Trialists' Collaborative Group (EBCTCG) conducted a meta-analysis of several randomized trials comparing different adjuvant chemotherapy regimens. They concluded that standard chemotherapies such as cyclophosphamide/methotrexate/5-fluorouracil (CMF) and standard AC reduced 8-year breast cancer mortality rates by 20–25%. The use of a more intense regimen combining anthracycline and taxane further reduced breast cancer mortality by 15–20%. However, despite being a small group, patients older than 70 years appeared to have had as great a reduction as younger women in breast cancer recurrence and mortality [55].

Anthracyclines such as doxorubicin and epirubicin are among the most active chemotherapeutic agents in breast cancer. However, their use in elderly patients is limited by cardiotoxicity. Given the risk of cardiotoxicity and multiple side effects from polychemotherapy, several anthracycline-sparing regimens have been tried in elderly TNBC patients, but none have become standard of care for several reasons.

In Cancer and Leukemia Group B (CALGB) 49,907 study, 633 patients aged >65 years with node-positive or high-risk node-negative early-stage breast cancer were randomized to standard polychemotherapy regimens such as AC and CMF versus capecitabine monotherapy [17]. At the median follow-up of 2.4 years, the risk of relapse and death in the capecitabine group was found to be twofold higher compared to the polychemotherapy group. In the subgroup analysis, HR-negative tumors seemed to benefit more from polychemotherapy, further establishing the principle that fit elderly patients with aggressive disease should not be undertreated.

Investigational Chemotherapy for Elderly patients (ICE) study was a prospective, multicenter, randomized phase III intergroup study comparing the outcome of patients of ≥65 years with or without adjuvant capecitabine treatment [56]. Elderly patients with early breast cancer with node-positive disease irrespective of additional risk factors or node-negative disease with at least one other risk factor, such as histologic tumor size ≥ 2 cm, grade 2 or 3, and ER- and PR-negative, received the bisphosphonate ibandronate with or without capecitabine. The primary endpoint was to compare DFS between the two treatments. About 14% of patients were triple-negative. The study did not show benefit of capecitabine monotherapy, and the 5-year invasive DFS was 78.8% vs. 75%, respectively. The results from this study, taken together with CALGB 49907, which already demonstrates superiority of polychemotherapy (AC and CMF) over capecitabine, support the use of the former in elderly patients with high-risk disease wherever feasible.

In the ICE II trial, the compliance with and toxicity of a combination of nab-paclitaxel and capecitabine (nPX) was compared to the combination of epirubicin and cyclophosphamide (EC) or CMF in an elderly population [57]. Although nPX is an anthracycline-sparing regimen, it was found to be poorly tolerated in elderly patients with higher incidence of deaths (5 vs. 1 in EC/CMF) and non-hematological toxicities (hand-foot syndrome, diarrhea, sensory neuropathy, and infections) (58.5% vs. 18.7%; $P < 0.001$). Grade 3–5 hematological toxicity was generally more frequent with EC/CMF (90.9% vs. 64.8%; $P < 0.001$). At a median follow-up of 22.8 months, there was no difference in OS or DFS in both arms. There was greater treatment discontinuation rate with the nPX arm.

In the phase II Elderly Docetaxel Adjuvant (ELDA) trial, women aged 65–79 years, at high risk of recurrence, were randomized to CMF versus weekly docetaxel [58]. A quarter of the study population was triple-negative. Single-agent docetaxel was not superior to CMF, and it was associated with worse quality of life.

Docetaxel and cyclophosphamide (TC) combination was studied as a non-anthracycline option in breast cancer in the US Oncology Research Trial 9735 where it was found to improve OS and DFS compared to 3-weekly AC [59]. The reported rates of grade 3 or 4 neutropenia were 61%, and the rate of febrile neutropenia in this trial was 4% in patients under 65 years and 8% in older than 65 years of age. Given the hematologic toxicity, the treatment completion rate in elderly is reported to be lower compared to younger populations (71% vs. 90%) despite use of prophylactic granulocyte colony-stimulating factor (GCSF) [60]. Moreover, in the recently published ABC trials, TC was reported to have inferior invasive DFS compared to taxane and anthracycline combination in TNBC patients [61]. Nevertheless, TC may be used as an anthracycline-sparing regimen in elderly patients who are at a high risk of cardiac toxicity.

CMF is a well-tolerated adjuvant chemotherapy option in elderly patients. There is evidence of efficacy in TNBC. In a Korean study for early-stage breast cancer, node-negative, T1–T2, 5-year OS with CMF was comparable to AC and CAF regimens (95.9%, 95.3%, and 95.9%, for AC, FAC, and CMF, respectively) [62]. CMF was shown to improve DFS in node-negative early TNBC when compared to the observation cohort. In the subgroup analysis of the tumors greater than 2 cm, the CMF group had significantly better DFS than the observation group (hazard ratio = 0.38, $P = 0.02$) [63]. CMF may be less efficacious in the larger, node-positive, TNBC when compared to anthracycline/taxane combinations; however, it is a reasonable option for elderly patients presenting with early-stage TNBC, given its favorable toxicity profile [64].

Capecitabine maintenance therapy may have found a new role in a subset of breast cancer patients who did not achieve pathological complete response with neoadjuvant anthracycline and taxane-based chemotherapy in the recently reported CREATE-X trial. In this trial, 910 patients with HER2-negative disease with residual invasive cancer after neoadjuvant chemotherapy were randomized to 6 months of capecitabine versus no further chemotherapy. At 5 years, the primary endpoint of DFS was 74.1% with capecitabine compared to 67.7% in the no further treatment arm (one-sided $P = 0.00524$). Overall survival rates were 89.2% and 83.9%

(one-sided $P < 0.01$). The HR-negative subgroup experienced a 42% reduction in risk with capecitabine treatment [65].

In summary, the approach to adjuvant treatment in TNBC should be individualized and take into account both patient and tumor-specific factors. For early-stage, node-negative breast cancers, regimens like TC and CMF seem appropriate if the patient is unable to tolerate anthracycline and taxane combinations. However, for locally advanced and node-positive tumors, the latter are still considered the standard of care. If there is a contraindication to receive anthracycline regimens, TC or CMF may be considered, as they still improve DFS and OS compared to no chemotherapy.

11.6   Use of Anthracyclines in the Elderly

Anthracyclines are the most effective chemotherapy agents in breast cancer. Elderly women with high-risk disease also derive benefit from anthracycline therapy [66–69]. However, there is a concern of higher cardiac toxicity in this population [70]. Cumulative destruction of myocytes is responsible for anthracycline-induced cardiomyopathy which is usually irreversible [71]. In the SEER analysis of elderly women treated with anthracyclines, patients between 65 and 70 years of age had a higher incidence of developing congestive heart failure at a 5-year follow-up compared to patients treated with other or no chemotherapy (19% versus 18% and 15%, respectively) [72]. Upon further follow-up of additional 5 years, these effects were accentuated. Comorbidities such as diabetes, coronary artery disease, and hypertension were significantly predictive of CHF in this and in prior studies. Interestingly, the group between 71 and 80 years of age did not have cardiotoxicity that differed by choice of treatment which suggests that it may be premature to not offer anthracycline-based treatment to elderly patients with aggressive disease [73].

11.7   Neoadjuvant Chemotherapy

Neoadjuvant chemotherapy (NAC), also referred to as preoperative or primary chemotherapy, refers to chemotherapy administered prior to tumor resection. Although preoperative chemotherapy has not been shown to improve DFS and OS for breast cancer when compared to postoperative therapy in operable patients, it helps in downstaging existing breast tumor, thereby increasing chances of breast conservation. Achievement of pathological complete response (pCR) defined as absence of any residual invasive tumor, if achieved, is an important predictor of superior DFS and OS. Anthracycline/taxane chemotherapy-based regimens have routinely been used in the neoadjuvant setting for TNBC with pCR ranging between 20 and 34% [74, 75]. Since TNBCs often harbor *BRCA1* mutations, the use of a platinum agent may be of special use in this setting. High pCR rates have been demonstrated with single-agent cisplatin in the neoadjuvant setting in *BRCA1*-mutated TNBC patients [76–78]. Two studies have evaluated the role of neoadjuvant carboplatin in TNBC.

In the GeparSixto trial, addition of carboplatin to doxorubicin/paclitaxel resulted in an increased pCR rate (53.2% with carboplatin and 36.9% without, $P = 0.005$). At 3 years, DFS was improved with addition of carboplatin (3-year DFS, 85.5% versus 76.1%, $P = 0.035$). Only 3% of patients in the study were >70 years of age [79]. In the CALGB 40603 trial, carboplatin or bevacizumab or both were added to the standard anthracycline and paclitaxel arm [80]. Addition of either agent showed improvement in pCR rate; however, specific treatment effect of carboplatin on EFS could not be demonstrated. Patients who achieved pCR had improved event-free survival in this study. Again, only 2% of the study population was >70 years of age. Patients in the carboplatin arm experienced greater hematologic toxicity.

The role of carboplatin in neoadjuvant chemotherapy remains unclear given these conflicting data. There may be a way to better select patient population likely to benefit from neoadjuvant carboplatin. Genetic defects in homologous recombination pathway as in the germline *BRCA1/2*-mutated tumors may render them uniquely susceptible to platinum-based therapy. In the subgroup analysis of GeparSixto trial, 70% of TNBC were found to have homologous recombination deficiency (HRD) [81]. Presence of HRD was a predictor of higher pCR rates (55.9% in HRD group vs. 29.9% in non-HRD) regardless of carboplatin. Addition of carboplatin to the HRD group further improved pCR rates from 45.2% to 64.9%. Given the lack of improvement in OS, there is no convincing data that these improved pCR rates translate into improved future outcomes.

11.8   Treatment of Metastatic Disease

Despite many advances in treatment options, metastatic breast cancer still remains an incurable disease. The purpose of chemotherapy in such a situation is prolongation of life and palliation of symptoms caused by cancer. Chemotherapy is recommended in elderly women with TNBC. There is no ideal sequence of treatments that can be applied to all patients [82]. In elderly patients, there is a preference for monotherapy, especially if the disease burden is limited given better toxicity profile and no difference in overall survival [83].

11.9   Individual Systemic Agents Available in the Metastatic Setting

11.9.1 Anthracyclines

Anthracyclines also retain their cardiotoxic properties when used in the metastatic setting. However, there are potentially lesser cardiotoxic formulations such as pegylated liposomal doxorubicin which have equal efficacy as doxorubicin [84, 85]. For older women who will receive an anthracycline, a baseline study for the cardiac left ventricular ejection fraction (LVEF) should be obtained prior to the initiation of treatment. In addition, symptoms should be carefully monitored and LVEF reassessed with onset of symptoms or periodically during therapy as per the guidelines endorsed by the American Heart Association/American College of Cardiology in conjunction with the American Society for Nuclear Cardiology and the American Society for Echocardiography [86, 87].

11.9.2 Taxanes

Besides anthracyclines, taxanes are one of the most active cytotoxic agents in the treatment of breast cancer and provide tumor response and survival benefit in elderly patients when used both in the first- or second-line metastatic setting [88]. With hypoalbuminemia associated with old age as well as reduced cytochrome P450 activity, the concentration of these drugs may increase in the body, predisposing to increased toxicity [89]. Studies have shown increased neurotoxicity from paclitaxel in patients who are older than 65 years of age [90]. Certain regimens like 3-weekly docetaxel are associated with high risk of hematological toxicity in elderly patients. In contrast, weekly docetaxel and weekly paclitaxel are well tolerated with less suppressive effects on the bone marrow. However, there is greater peripheral neuropathy associated with weekly paclitaxel and severe fatigue in weekly docetaxel [91–94]. Both weekly paclitaxel and docetaxel regimens have been compared in a randomized trial of 70 metastatic breast cancer patients, with 28 patients aged >70 showing median OS data favoring weekly paclitaxel (56 versus 32 weeks) [95].

There is limited data regarding the use of nanoparticle albumin-bound paclitaxel (nab-paclitaxel) in elderly patients with breast cancer. When compared to 3-weekly paclitaxel, 3-weekly nab-paclitaxel has superior tumor response rate and progression-free survival (PFS) advantage in advanced breast cancer. The incidence of neuropathy with 3-weekly nab-paclitaxel is greater than what has been reported with weekly paclitaxel. In this trial, nab-paclitaxel-associated neuropathy required a shorter time period to resolve compared to paclitaxel neuropathy [96, 97].

Although there has been no head-to-head comparison between single-agent nab-paclitaxel and paclitaxel, in a phase III clinical trial combining bevacizumab with nab-paclitaxel, paclitaxel, or ixabepilone, respectively, in chemo-naïve population, superiority of the former agent could not be demonstrated. Ixabepilone, which is a semisynthetic analogue of epothilone B, is found to be inferior to paclitaxel. There was significantly worse neuropathy in the nab-paclitaxel arm [98].

11.9.3 Capecitabine

Capecitabine is an efficacious, oral option for elderly patients with metastatic breast cancer [99]. Although capecitabine has been approved by the Food and Drug Administration (FDA) as a 2-week on and 1-week off schedule, this method of administration has associated toxicities such as hand-foot syndrome, mucositis, and diarrhea, which often require dose reduction [100, 101]. Traina and colleagues worked on a mathematical model to optimize therapeutic dosing based on the

Simon-Norton model, which determines treatment schedule based on efficacy rather than toxicity. They demonstrated that capecitabine schedule with 7 days of treatment followed by 7 days of rest (7–7) will improve efficacy and minimize toxicity [102–104]. Although feasible, combination of capecitabine with other agents has a modest effect on efficacy [105–107].

11.9.4 Eribulin

Eribulin was FDA approved for MBC after it demonstrated good responses in heavily pretreated patients in a large phase III trial with a 2.7-month improvement in OS (HR, 0.81; 95% CI, 0.68-0.96, 0.014) [108]. In a pooled analysis of 827 patients with metastatic breast cancer treated with eribulin on a 21-day cycle, patients were divided into four age groups: <50 years, 50–59 years, 60–69 years, and >70 years. It was found that overall response rate (ORR) as well as overall and progression-free survival was similar across all age groups. Older cohort experienced greater peripheral edema, fatigue, and dizziness, while the younger cohort reported greater nausea and vomiting. The rates of neutropenia, febrile neutropenia, leukopenia, peripheral neuropathy, alopecia, and dyspnea were similar across all age groups. The efficacy of eribulin in heavily pretreated patients coupled with manageable toxicity profile shows that the elderly fit patients with triple-negative metastatic breast cancer can derive equal benefit from eribulin compared to their younger counterparts [108–111].

11.9.5 Vinorelbine

There are some data that show variable pharmacokinetics of vinorelbine related to age [112, 113]. However, another study demonstrated that vinorelbine clearance was affected by hepatic and renal function and not by age [114]. In a phase II study of women >60 years of age with metastatic breast cancer, response rate with vinorelbine was 38%. However, with conventional weekly dose of 30 mg/m², vinorelbine caused grade 3 or 4 neutropenia in 8% of the study population, requiring dose reduction to 20 mg/m² [115, 116].

11.9.6 Platinum Agents

The role of platinum agents in metastatic TNBC is unclear. Trials in unselected patients show marginal improvement in PFS with no improvement in OS [117, 118]. However, in a trial of single-agent cisplatin compared to the standard arm of single-agent taxane, treatment with cisplatin nearly doubled the objective response rate (68% vs. 33.3%, $P = 0.003$) and PFS (6.8 months vs. 3.1 months) in patients with germline BRCA mutation only [119]. Early efforts to selectively target *BRCA*-mutated tumors focused on impaired homologous repair and inability to repair DNA cross-links caused by platinum salts [120]. Gemcitabine and carboplatin is another regimen which has shown clinical efficacy with ORR (PR+ SD) of 64% [121, 122]. As in the neoadjuvant setting, it is important to further identify the subset of TNBCs such as those that harbor a germline *BRCA* mutation or have a HRD, who can specifically benefit from the addition of platinum agents.

11.9.7 Poly(ADP-ribose) Polymerase Inhibitors

Triple-negative breast cancers often harbor mutations in *BRCA1/2* genes. The normal *BRCA1/2* genes code for proteins that play a role in the repair of DNA double-strand breaks by homologous recombination. Therefore, *BRCA*-mutated breast cancers have defective DNA repair by homologous recombination, and the use of alternative DNA-repair mechanisms, which are error prone, can lead to accumulation of genetic aberrations, leading to tumorigenesis. Synthetic lethality can be introduced by further inhibiting single-stranded DNA repair by poly(ADP-ribose) polymerase (PARP) inhibitors [123]. In the recently published phase III OlympiAD study, the PARP inhibitor olaparib demonstrated statistically significant, clinically meaningful benefit in patients with germline *BRCA*-mutated HER2-negative breast cancers when compared to treatment of physician's choice, with a 3-month improvement in PFS and doubling of ORR (29% vs. 60%). It was well tolerated with low treatment discontinuation rates and prolonged time to deterioration of health-related quality of life [124].

11.9.8 Immunotherapy

There is a growing interest in analyzing the role of immunomodulatory agents in management of TNBC. Programmed death-1 (PD-1) receptor is expressed on activated T cells and limits autoimmune response to inflammatory stimuli. PDL-1 is a ligand of PD-1 immunosuppressive signal that is upregulated in response to pro-inflammatory ligands such as interferon-gamma. PDL-1 is expressed on several cancers and may play a major role in PD-1 pathway inhibition [125–128]. PDL1 is expressed in about 20–30% of TNBC [129]. Higher PDL-1 mRNA expression was demonstrated in the TNBC versus non-TNBC in the Cancer Genome Atlas Network [130]. In a phase I study of heavily pretreated TNBC whose tumors expressed PDL-1, pembrolizumab was able to produce durable responses in 18.4% of patients ranging from 15 to >47.3 weeks (median not reached) [131]. Median age of patients enrolled in this study was younger (50.5, range: 29–72). The grade 2 side effects included anemia, pyrexia, aseptic meningitis, and colitis. There was one treatment-related death due to disseminated intravascular coagulation (DIC). There is limited data on efficacy and tolerability of immunotherapy in elderly patients.

Atezolizumab is a humanized monoclonal antibody that inhibits binding of PD-L1 to PD-1 and B7.2 and has demonstrated single-agent activity in metastatic TNBC. In a phase IB trial of 32 patients, the combination of atezolizumab and nab-paclitaxel resulted in an ORR of 41% across all lines of prior therapy, regardless of PD-L1 status [132]. In the phase III IMpassion130 trial, patients with previously untreated metastatic TNBC will be randomized to nab-paclitaxel plus placebo or nab-paclitaxel plus atezolizumab. The primary endpoint of the study is PFS in the full population and in a PD-L1-positive group. Secondary endpoints include OS, ORR, and duration of response. The target enrollment goal for the trial is 350 patients (NCT02425891).

11.9.9 Androgen Receptor Inhibition

AR receptor expression is found in about 30% of TNBC [133]. A subset of TNBC expressing androgen receptors may benefit from therapies that inhibit AR signaling pathway. In the first multicenter phase II trial of bicalutamide in patients with metastatic TNBC who had >10% nuclear expression of AR, clinical benefit rate (complete response [CR]+ partial response [PR]+ stable disease [SD]) was 19% with median PFS of 12 weeks. However, a subset of patients demonstrated prolonged responses, ranging in years. Enzalutamide is an orally administered pure androgen receptor signaling inhibitor and has shown efficacy in metastatic TNBC. A phase II trial enrolled 118 women with AR-positive TNBC patients who were treated with 160 mg of enzalutamide PO daily until disease progression. The trial met its primary endpoint of clinical benefit at 16 weeks of therapy. Of the 75 patients who could be evaluated, 35% achieved a clinical benefit (two CRs and seven PRs). The clinical benefit rate at ≥24 weeks was 29%. The median PFS was 14.7 weeks [134]. The ENDEAR (A Phase III, Randomized, International Study Comparing the Efficacy and Safety of Enzalutamide in Combination with Paclitaxel Chemotherapy or as Monotherapy Versus Placebo with Paclitaxel in Patients with Advanced, Diagnostic-Positive, Triple-Negative Breast Cancer) (NCT02929576) trial will evaluate the efficacy and safety of enzalutamide in combination with paclitaxel chemotherapy or as monotherapy versus placebo with paclitaxel in patients with locally advanced or metastatic TNBC whose tumors test positive for a novel gene expression profile, which is referred to as diagnostic-positive TNBC. Overall, antiandrogens are well tolerated with main side effects being fatigue and anorexia. There have been no serious side effects reported. Hence, they may be a useful option in elderly population when comorbidities preclude them from getting aggressive chemotherapy regimens.

Conclusion

Although TNBC is a disease of the young, about 18% of patients with TNBC are >65 years of age. However, patients in the elderly age group are often undertreated due to fear of toxicity and underlying comorbidities. Data shows that when appropriately prescribed, elderly patients derive the same benefits from systemic therapies as their younger counterparts. Appropriate geriatric assessment tools should be employed when prescribing systemic therapies to these patients.

References

1. Ferlay J, Soerjomataram I, Dikshit R, Eser S, Mathers C, Rebelo M, Parkin DM, Forman D, Bray F. Cancer incidence and mortality worldwide: sources, methods and major patterns in GLOBOCAN 2012. Int J Cancer. 2015;136(5):E359–86. https://doi.org/10.1002/ijc.29210. PMID:25220842 Published online 9 October 2014.
2. Carlson RW, et al. NCCN Task Force Report: breast cancer in the older woman. J Natl Compr Canc Netw. 2008;6(Suppl 4): S1–25; quiz S26–7.
3. Perou CM, et al. Molecular portraits of human breast tumours. Nature. 2000;406(6797):747–52.
4. Dent R, et al. Triple-negative breast cancer: clinical features and patterns of recurrence. Clin Cancer Res. 2007;13(15 Pt 1):4429–34.
5. Liedtke C, et al. Response to neoadjuvant therapy and long-term survival in patients with triple-negative breast cancer. J Clin Oncol. 2008;26(8):1275–81.
6. Bauer KR, et al. Descriptive analysis of estrogen receptor (ER)-negative, progesterone receptor (PR)-negative, and HER2-negative invasive breast cancer, the so-called triple-negative phenotype: a population-based study from the California cancer Registry. Cancer. 2007;109(9):1721–8.
7. Mandelblatt JS, et al. Patient and physician decision styles and breast cancer chemotherapy use in older women: Cancer and Leukemia Group B protocol 369901. J Clin Oncol. 2012;30(21):2609–14.
8. Ring A, et al. The treatment of early breast cancer in women over the age of 70. Br J Cancer. 2011;105(2):189–93.
9. Konigsberg R, et al. Tumor characteristics and recurrence patterns in triple negative breast cancer: a comparison between younger (<65) and elderly (>/=65) patients. Eur J Cancer. 2012;48(16):2962–8.
10. Cancello G, et al. Prognosis in women with small (T1mic,T1a,T1b) node-negative operable breast cancer by immunohistochemically selected subtypes. Breast Cancer Res Treat. 2011;127(3):713–20.
11. Gangi A, et al. Breast-conserving therapy for triple-negative breast cancer. JAMA Surg. 2014;149(3):252–8.
12. Lowery AJ, et al. Locoregional recurrence after breast cancer surgery: a systematic review by receptor phenotype. Breast Cancer Res Treat. 2012;133(3):831–41.
13. Liedtke C, et al. The prognostic impact of age in patients with triple-negative breast cancer. Breast Cancer Res Treat. 2013;138(2):591–9.
14. Zhu W, et al. Age-related disparity in immediate prognosis of patients with triple-negative breast cancer: a population-based study from SEER Cancer Registries. PLoS One. 2015;10(5):e0128345.
15. Hutchins LF, et al. Underrepresentation of patients 65 years of age or older in cancer-treatment trials. N Engl J Med. 1999;341(27):2061–7.
16. Freedman RA, et al. Accrual of older patients with breast cancer to alliance systemic therapy trials over time: protocol A151527. J Clin Oncol. 2017;35(4):421–31.
17. Muss HB, et al. Adjuvant chemotherapy in older women with early-stage breast cancer. N Engl J Med. 2009;360(20):2055–65.
18. Gibreel WO, et al. Mastectomy and immediate breast reconstruction for cancer in the elderly: a National Cancer Data Base Study. J Am Coll Surg. 2017;224(5):895–905.
19. Hughes KS, et al. Lumpectomy plus tamoxifen with or without irradiation in women age 70 years or older with early breast cancer: long-term follow-up of CALGB 9343. J Clin Oncol. 2013;31(19):2382–7.
20. Kunkler IH, et al. Breast-conserving surgery with or without irradiation in women aged 65 years or older with early breast cancer (PRIME II): a randomised controlled trial. Lancet Oncol. 2015;16(3):266–73.
21. Hatch SS. Outcomes associated with adjuvant radiation after lumpectomy for elderly women with T1-2N0M0 triple-negative breast cancer: SEER analysis. J Clin Oncol. 2015;33(28_Suppl):39.

22. Extermann M, Balducci L, Lyman GH. What threshold for adjuvant therapy in older breast cancer patients? J Clin Oncol. 2000;18(8):1709–17.
23. Singh JC, Lichtman SM. Effect of age on drug metabolism in women with breast cancer. Expert Opin Drug Metab Toxicol. 2015;11(5):757–66.
24. Hershman DL, Shao T. Anthracycline cardiotoxicity after breast cancer treatment. Oncology (Williston Park). 2009;23(3):227–34.
25. Von Hoff DD, Rozencweig M, Piccart M. The cardiotoxicity of anticancer agents. Semin Oncol. 1982;9(1):23–33.
26. Venook AP, et al. Phase I and pharmacokinetic trial of paclitaxel in patients with hepatic dysfunction: Cancer and Leukemia Group B 9264. J Clin Oncol. 1998;16(5):1811–9.
27. Venook AP, et al. Phase I and pharmacokinetic trial of gemcitabine in patients with hepatic or renal dysfunction: Cancer and Leukemia Group B 9565. J Clin Oncol. 2000;18(14):2780–7.
28. Venook AP, et al. A phase I and pharmacokinetic study of irinotecan in patients with hepatic or renal dysfunction or with prior pelvic radiation: CALGB 9863. Ann Oncol. 2003;14(12):1783–90.
29. Lichtman SM, Skirvin JA, Vemulapalli S. Pharmacology of antineoplastic agents in older cancer patients. Crit Rev Oncol Hematol. 2003;46(2):101–14.
30. Lichtman SM, et al. International Society of Geriatric Oncology Chemotherapy Taskforce: evaluation of chemotherapy in older patients—an analysis of the medical literature. J Clin Oncol. 2007;25(14):1832–43.
31. Yuen GJ. Altered pharmacokinetics in the elderly. Clin Geriatr Med. 1990;6(2):257–67.
32. Baker SD, Grochow LB. Pharmacology of cancer chemotherapy in the older person. Clin Geriatr Med. 1997;13(1):169–83.
33. Neugut AI, et al. Association between prescription co-payment amount and compliance with adjuvant hormonal therapy in women with early-stage breast cancer. J Clin Oncol. 2011;29(18):2534–42.
34. Partridge AH, et al. Adherence and persistence with oral adjuvant chemotherapy in older women with early-stage breast cancer in CALGB 49907: adherence companion study 60104. J Clin Oncol. 2010;28(14):2418–22.
35. Partridge AH, et al. Nonadherence to adjuvant tamoxifen therapy in women with primary breast cancer. J Clin Oncol. 2003;21(4):602–6.
36. Maggiore RJ, et al. Polypharmacy and potentially inappropriate medication use in older adults with cancer undergoing chemotherapy: effect on chemotherapy-related toxicity and hospitalization during treatment. J Am Geriatr Soc. 2014;62(8):1505–12.
37. Lichtman SM, Boparai MK. Anticancer drug therapy in the older cancer patient: pharmacology and polypharmacy. Curr Treat Options Oncol. 2008;9(2–3):191–203.
38. Salazar JA, Poon I, Nair M. Clinical consequences of polypharmacy in elderly: expect the unexpected, think the unthinkable. Expert Opin Drug Saf. 2007;6(6):695–704.
39. Sparreboom A, et al. Herbal remedies in the United States: potential adverse interactions with anticancer agents. J Clin Oncol. 2004;22(12):2489–503.
40. Maggiore RJ, et al. Use of complementary medications among older adults with cancer. Cancer. 2012;118(19):4815–23.
41. Puts MT, et al. A systematic review of factors influencing older adults' decision to accept or decline cancer treatment. Cancer Treat Rev. 2015;41(2):197–215.
42. Barcenas CH, et al. Anthracycline regimen adherence in older patients with early breast cancer. Oncologist. 2012;17(3):303–11.
43. de Glas NA, et al. Validity of adjuvant! Online program in older patients with breast cancer: a population-based study. Lancet Oncol. 2014;15(7):722–9.
44. Pal SK, Katheria V, Hurria A. Evaluating the older patient with cancer: understanding frailty and the geriatric assessment. CA Cancer J Clin. 2010;60(2):120–32.
45. Wildiers H, et al. International Society of Geriatric Oncology consensus on geriatric assessment in older patients with cancer. J Clin Oncol. 2014;32(24):2595–603.
46. Version, N.C.C.N.N.O.A.O., A.a. http://www.nccn.org/professionals/physician_gls/pdf/senior, and pdf. Accessed June 20.

47. Extermann M, et al. Predicting the risk of chemotherapy toxicity in older patients: the Chemotherapy Risk Assessment Scale for High-Age Patients (CRASH) score. Cancer. 2012;118(13):3377–86.
48. Hurria A, et al. Developing a cancer-specific geriatric assessment: a feasibility study. Cancer. 2005;104(9):1998–2005.
49. Hurria A, et al. Predicting chemotherapy toxicity in older adults with cancer: a prospective multicenter study. J Clin Oncol. 2011;29(25):3457–65.
50. Hurria A, et al. Validation of a prediction tool for chemotherapy toxicity in older adults with cancer. J Clin Oncol. 2016;34(20):2366–71.
51. Jolly TA, et al. Geriatric assessment-identified deficits in older cancer patients with normal performance status. Oncologist. 2015;20(4):379–85.
52. Kaplan HG, Malmgren JA, Atwood MK. Adjuvant chemotherapy and differential invasive breast cancer specific survival in elderly women. J Geriatr Oncol. 2013;4(2):148–56.
53. Leonard R, et al. Adjuvant chemotherapy in older women (ACTION) study—what did we learn from the pilot phase? Br J Cancer. 2011;105(9):1260–6.
54. Karavasilis V, et al. Safety and tolerability of anthracycline-containing adjuvant chemotherapy in elderly high-risk breast cancer patients. Clin Breast Cancer. 2016;16(4):291–298 e3.
55. Early Breast Cancer Trialists' Collaborative, G., et al. Comparisons between different polychemotherapy regimens for early breast cancer: meta-analyses of long-term outcome among 100,000 women in 123 randomised trials. Lancet. 2012;379(9814):432–44.
56. von Minckwitz G, Reimer T, Potenberg J, et al. The phase III ICE study: adjuvant ibandronate with or without capecitabine in elderly patients with moderate or high risk early breast cancer. In: San Antonio breast cancer symposium. Abstract S3-04. Presented December 11, 2014. 2014.
57. von Minckwitz G, et al. A randomized phase 2 study comparing EC or CMF versus nab-paclitaxel plus capecitabine as adjuvant chemotherapy for nonfrail elderly patients with moderate to high-risk early breast cancer (ICE II-GBG 52). Cancer. 2015;121(20):3639–48.
58. Perrone F, et al. Weekly docetaxel versus CMF as adjuvant chemotherapy for older women with early breast cancer: final results of the randomized phase III ELDA trial. Ann Oncol. 2015;26(4):675–82.
59. Jones S, et al. Docetaxel with cyclophosphamide is associated with an overall survival benefit compared with doxorubicin and cyclophosphamide: 7-year follow-up of US Oncology Research Trial 9735. J Clin Oncol. 2009;27(8):1177–83.
60. Ngamphaiboon N, et al. Febrile neutropenia in adjuvant docetaxel and cyclophosphamide (TC) with prophylactic pegfilgrastim in breast cancer patients: a retrospective analysis. Med Oncol. 2012;29(3):1495–501.
61. Blum JL, et al. Anthracyclines in early breast cancer: the ABC trials-USOR 06-090, NSABP B-46-I/USOR 07132, and NSABP B-49 (NRG Oncology). J Clin Oncol. 2017;35(23):2647–55.
62. Kim HA, et al. Evaluation of the survival benefit of different chemotherapy regimens in patients with T1-2N0 triple-negative breast cancer. J Breast Cancer. 2015;18(3):271–8.
63. Wu CE, et al. Identification of patients with node-negative, triple-negative breast cancer who benefit from adjuvant cyclophosphamide, methotrexate, and 5-fluorouracil chemotherapy. Anticancer Res. 2014;34(3):1301–6.
64. Kadakia A, et al. CMF-regimen preferred as first-course chemotherapy for older and sicker women with breast cancer: findings from a SEER-Medicare-based population study. Am J Clin Oncol. 2015;38(2):165–73.
65. Masuda N, et al. Adjuvant capecitabine for breast cancer after preoperative chemotherapy. N Engl J Med. 2017;376(22):2147–59.
66. Ibrahim NK, et al. Doxorubicin-based adjuvant chemotherapy in elderly breast cancer patients: the M.D. Anderson experience, with long-term follow-up. Ann Oncol. 2000;11(12):1597–601.
67. Muss HB, et al. Adjuvant chemotherapy in older and younger women with lymph node-positive breast cancer. JAMA. 2005;293(9):1073–81.

68. Elkin EB, et al. Adjuvant chemotherapy and survival in older women with hormone receptor-negative breast cancer: assessing outcome in a population-based, observational cohort. J Clin Oncol. 2006;24(18):2757–64.
69. Downey LB. Adjuvant treatment of breast cancer in the elderly. Understanding and addressing the challenges. Oncology (Williston Park). 2008;22(3):286–93; discussion 297–8.
70. Fumoleau P, et al. Long-term cardiac toxicity after adjuvant epirubicin-based chemotherapy in early breast cancer: French Adjuvant Study Group results. Ann Oncol. 2006;17(1):85–92.
71. Ewer MS, Lenihan DJ. Left ventricular ejection fraction and cardiotoxicity: is our ear really to the ground? J Clin Oncol. 2008;26(8):1201–3.
72. Hershman DL, et al. Doxorubicin, cardiac risk factors, and cardiac toxicity in elderly patients with diffuse B-cell non-Hodgkin's lymphoma. J Clin Oncol. 2008;26(19):3159–65.
73. Pinder MC, et al. Congestive heart failure in older women treated with adjuvant anthracycline chemotherapy for breast cancer. J Clin Oncol. 2007;25(25):3808–15.
74. Huober J, et al. Effect of neoadjuvant anthracycline-taxane-based chemotherapy in different biological breast cancer phenotypes: overall results from the GeparTrio study. Breast Cancer Res Treat. 2010;124(1):133–40.
75. Oakman C, Viale G, Di Leo A. Management of triple negative breast cancer. Breast. 2010;19(5):312–21.
76. Byrski T, et al. Pathologic complete response rates in young women with BRCA1-positive breast cancers after neoadjuvant chemotherapy. J Clin Oncol. 2010;28(3):375–9.
77. Byrski T, et al. Response to neoadjuvant therapy with cisplatin in BRCA1-positive breast cancer patients. Breast Cancer Res Treat. 2009;115(2):359–63.
78. Byrski T, et al. Pathologic complete response to neoadjuvant cisplatin in BRCA1-positive breast cancer patients. Breast Cancer Res Treat. 2014;147(2):401–5.
79. von Minckwitz G, Loibl S, Schneeweiss A, Salat C, Rezai M, Zahm D-M, et al. Abstract S2-04: early survival analysis of the randomized phase II trial investigating the addition of carboplatin to neoadjuvant therapy for triplenegative and HER2-positive early breast cancer (GeparSixto). Cancer Res. 2016;76:S2–4.
80. Sikov WM, et al. Impact of the addition of carboplatin and/or bevacizumab to neoadjuvant once-per-week paclitaxel followed by dose-dense doxorubicin and cyclophosphamide on pathologic complete response rates in stage II to III triple-negative breast cancer: CALGB 40603 (Alliance). J Clin Oncol. 2015;33(1):13–21.
81. von Minckwitz G, Timms K, Untch M, et al. Prediction ofpathological complete response (pCR) by homologous recombination deficiency (HRD) after carboplatin-containing neo-adjuvant chemotherapy in patients with TNBC: results from GeparSixto. J Clin Oncol. 2015;33:abstr 1004.
82. Kaufman PA, et al. Phase III open-label randomized study of eribulin mesylate versus capecitabine in patients with locally advanced or metastatic breast cancer previously treated with an anthracycline and a taxane. J Clin Oncol. 2015;33(6):594–601.
83. Dear RF, et al. Combination versus sequential single agent chemotherapy for metastatic breast cancer. Cochrane Database Syst Rev. 2013;(12):CD008792.
84. Coleman RE, et al. A randomised phase II study of two different schedules of pegylated liposomal doxorubicin in metastatic breast cancer (EORTC-10993). Eur J Cancer. 2006;42(7):882–7.
85. O'Brien ME, et al. Reduced cardiotoxicity and comparable efficacy in a phase III trial of pegylated liposomal doxorubicin HCl (CAELYX/Doxil) versus conventional doxorubicin for first-line treatment of metastatic breast cancer. Ann Oncol. 2004;15(3):440–9.
86. Cheitlin MD, et al. ACC/AHA/ASE 2003 guideline update for the clinical application of echocardiography: summary article. A report of the American College of Cardiology/American Heart Association Task Force on Practice Guidelines (ACC/AHA/ASE Committee to update the 1997 guidelines for the clinical application of echocardiography). J Am Soc Echocardiogr. 2003;16(10):1091–110.
87. Klocke FJ, et al. ACC/AHA/ASNC guidelines for the clinical use of cardiac radionuclide imaging—executive summary: a report of the American College of Cardiology/American

Heart Association Task Force on Practice Guidelines (ACC/AHA/ASNC Committee to revise the 1995 guidelines for the clinical use of cardiac radionuclide imaging). J Am Coll Cardiol. 2003;42(7):1318–33.

88. Yared JA, Tkaczuk KH. Update on taxane development: new analogs and new formulations. Drug Des Devel Ther. 2012;6:371–84.

89. Biganzoli L, et al. Taxanes in the treatment of breast cancer: have we better defined their role in older patients? A position paper from a SIOG Task Force. Cancer Treat Rev. 2016;43:19–26.

90. Lichtman SM, et al. Paclitaxel efficacy and toxicity in older women with metastatic breast cancer: combined analysis of CALGB 9342 and 9840. Ann Oncol. 2012;23(3):632–8.

91. Seidman AD, et al. Randomized phase III trial of weekly compared with every-3-weeks paclitaxel for metastatic breast cancer, with trastuzumab for all HER-2 overexpressors and random assignment to trastuzumab or not in HER-2 nonoverexpressors: final results of Cancer and Leukemia Group B protocol 9840. J Clin Oncol. 2008;26(10):1642–9.

92. ten Tije AJ, et al. Weekly paclitaxel as first-line chemotherapy for elderly patients with metastatic breast cancer. A multicentre phase II trial. Eur J Cancer. 2004;40(3):352–7.

93. Hainsworth JD, et al. Weekly docetaxel in the treatment of elderly patients with advanced breast cancer: a Minnie Pearl Cancer Research Network phase II trial. J Clin Oncol. 2001;19(15):3500–5.

94. Perez EA, et al. Weekly paclitaxel in women age 65 and above with metastatic breast cancer. Breast Cancer Res Treat. 2002;73(1):85–8.

95. Wildiers H, Paridaens R. Taxanes in elderly breast cancer patients. Cancer Treat Rev. 2004;30(4):333–42.

96. Gradishar WJ, et al. Significantly longer progression-free survival with nab-paclitaxel compared with docetaxel as first-line therapy for metastatic breast cancer. J Clin Oncol. 2009;27(22):3611–9.

97. Gradishar WJ, et al. Phase III trial of nanoparticle albumin-bound paclitaxel compared with polyethylated castor oil-based paclitaxel in women with breast cancer. J Clin Oncol. 2005;23(31):7794–803.

98. Rugo HS, et al. Randomized phase III trial of paclitaxel once per week compared with nanoparticle albumin-bound nab-paclitaxel once per week or ixabepilone with bevacizumab as first-line chemotherapy for locally recurrent or metastatic breast cancer: CALGB 40502/NCCTG N063H (Alliance). J Clin Oncol. 2015;33(21):2361–9.

99. Bajetta E, et al. Safety and efficacy of two different doses of capecitabine in the treatment of advanced breast cancer in older women. J Clin Oncol. 2005;23(10):2155–61.

100. Fumoleau P, et al. Multicentre, phase II study evaluating capecitabine monotherapy in patients with anthracycline- and taxane-pretreated metastatic breast cancer. Eur J Cancer. 2004;40(4):536–42.

101. Oshaughnessy JA, et al. Randomized, open-label, phase II trial of oral capecitabine (Xeloda) vs. a reference arm of intravenous CMF (cyclophosphamide, methotrexate and 5-fluorouracil) as first-line therapy for advanced/metastatic breast cancer. Ann Oncol. 2001;12(9):1247–54.

102. Traina TA, et al. Optimizing chemotherapy dose and schedule by Norton-Simon mathematical modeling. Breast Dis. 2010;31(1):7–18.

103. Traina TA, et al. Phase I study of a novel capecitabine schedule based on the Norton-Simon mathematical model in patients with metastatic breast cancer. J Clin Oncol. 2008;26(11):1797–802.

104. Hudis C, Traina T, Norton L. Capecitabine dosing is not yet optimized for breast cancer. Ann Oncol. 2010;21(11):2291; author reply 2291–2.

105. Traina TA, Theodoulou M, Dugan U, et al. A novel capecitabine dosing schedule combined with bevacizumab is safe and active in patients with metastatic breast cancer: a phase II study. J Clin Oncol (Meeting Abstracts). 2008;26(15Suppl):1101.

106. Welt A, et al. Capecitabine and bevacizumab with or without vinorelbine in first-line treatment of HER2/neu-negative metastatic or locally advanced breast cancer: final efficacy and safety data of the randomised, open-label superiority phase 3 CARIN trial. Breast Cancer Res Treat. 2016;156(1):97–107.

107. Wang J, et al. Capecitabine combined with docetaxel versus vinorelbine followed by capecitabine maintenance medication for first-line treatment of patients with advanced breast cancer: phase 3 randomized trial. Cancer. 2015;121(19):3412–21.
108. Cortes J, et al. Eribulin monotherapy versus treatment of physician's choice in patients with metastatic breast cancer (EMBRACE): a phase 3 open-label randomised study. Lancet. 2011;377(9769):914–23.
109. Cortes J, et al. Phase II study of the halichondrin B analog eribulin mesylate in patients with locally advanced or metastatic breast cancer previously treated with an anthracycline, a taxane, and capecitabine. J Clin Oncol. 2010;28(25):3922–8.
110. Vahdat LT, et al. Phase II study of eribulin mesylate, a halichondrin B analog, in patients with metastatic breast cancer previously treated with an anthracycline and a taxane. J Clin Oncol. 2009;27(18):2954–61.
111. Muss H, et al. Eribulin monotherapy in patients aged 70 years and older with metastatic breast cancer. Oncologist. 2014;19(4):318–27.
112. Gauvin A, et al. Bayesian estimate of vinorelbine pharmacokinetic parameters in elderly patients with advanced metastatic cancer. Clin Cancer Res. 2000;6(7):2690–5.
113. Sorio R, et al. Pharmacokinetics and tolerance of vinorelbine in elderly patients with metastatic breast cancer. Eur J Cancer. 1997;33(2):301–3.
114. Wong M, et al. Predictors of vinorelbine pharmacokinetics and pharmacodynamics in patients with cancer. J Clin Oncol. 2006;24(16):2448–55.
115. Baweja M, et al. Phase II trial of oral vinorelbine for the treatment of metastatic breast cancer in patients > or = 65 years of age: an NCCTG study. Ann Oncol. 2006;17(4):623–9.
116. Rossi A, et al. Single agent vinorelbine as first-line chemotherapy in elderly patients with advanced breast cancer. Anticancer Res. 2003;23(2C):1657–64.
117. Sirohi B, et al. Platinum-based chemotherapy in triple-negative breast cancer. Ann Oncol. 2008;19(11):1847–52.
118. Staudacher L, et al. Platinum-based chemotherapy in metastatic triple-negative breast cancer: the Institut Curie experience. Ann Oncol. 2011;22(4):848–56.
119. Tutt A, Cheang MCU, Kilburn L, et al. BRCA1 methylation status, silencing and treatment effect in the TNT trial: a randomized phase III trial of carboplatin compared with docetaxel for patients with metastatic or recurrent locally advanced triple negative or BRCA1/2 breast cancer (CRUK/07/012). Paper presented at 39th San Antonio breast cancer symposium; Dec 2016; San Antonio, TX.
120. Alli E, et al. Enhanced sensitivity to cisplatin and gemcitabine in Brca1-deficient murine mammary epithelial cells. BMC Pharmacol. 2011;11:7.
121. Loesch D, et al. Phase II trial of gemcitabine/carboplatin (plus trastuzumab in HER2-positive disease) in patients with metastatic breast cancer. Clin Breast Cancer. 2008;8(2):178–86.
122. Yardley DA, et al. A phase II trial of gemcitabine/carboplatin with or without trastuzumab in the first-line treatment of patients with metastatic breast cancer. Clin Breast Cancer. 2008;8(5):425–31.
123. Lord CJ, Tutt AN, Ashworth A. Synthetic lethality and cancer therapy: lessons learned from the development of PARP inhibitors. Annu Rev Med. 2015;66:455–70.
124. Robson M, et al. Olaparib for metastatic breast cancer in patients with a germline BRCA mutation. N Engl J Med. 2017;377(6):523–33.
125. Keir ME, et al. PD-1 and its ligands in tolerance and immunity. Annu Rev Immunol. 2008;26:677–704.
126. Nishimura H, et al. Developmentally regulated expression of the PD-1 protein on the surface of double-negative (CD4-CD8-) thymocytes. Int Immunol. 1996;8(5):773–80.
127. Pardoll DM. The blockade of immune checkpoints in cancer immunotherapy. Nat Rev Cancer. 2012;12(4):252–64.
128. Topalian SL, Drake CG, Pardoll DM. Targeting the PD-1/B7-H1(PD-L1) pathway to activate anti-tumor immunity. Curr Opin Immunol. 2012;24(2):207–12.
129. Mittendorf EA, et al. PD-L1 expression in triple-negative breast cancer. Cancer Immunol Res. 2014;2(4):361–70.

130. Cancer Genome Atlas, N. Comprehensive molecular portraits of human breast tumours. Nature. 2012;490(7418):61–70.
131. Nanda R, et al. Pembrolizumab in patients with advanced triple-negative breast cancer: phase Ib KEYNOTE-012 Study. J Clin Oncol. 2016;34(21):2460–7.
132. Adams S, Diamond J, Hamilton E, et al. Safety and clinical activity of atezolizumab (anti-PDL1) in combination with nab-paclitaxel in patients with metastatic triple-negative breast cancer. Presented at San Antonio breast cancer symposium; December 8–12, 2015; San Antonio, TX. Abstract P2-11-06; 2016.
133. Caiazza F, et al. Preclinical evaluation of the AR inhibitor enzalutamide in triple-negative breast cancer cells. Endocr Relat Cancer. 2016;23(4):323–34.
134. Tiffany A, Traina KM, Yardley DA, O'Shaughnessy J, et al. Results from a phase 2 study of enzalutamide (ENZA), an androgen receptor (AR) inhibitor, in advanced AR+ triple-negative breast cancer (TNBC). J Clin Oncol. 2015;33(suppl; abstr 1003):2015.